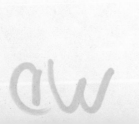

HEALTH CARE MANAGEMENT

A Contemporary Perspective

Seth B. Goldsmith
University of Massachusetts

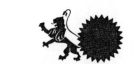

AN ASPEN PUBLICATION ®
Aspen Systems Corporation
Rockville, Maryland
London
1981

 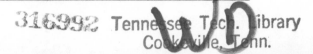

Library of Congress Cataloging in Publication Data

Goldsmith, Seth B.
Health care management.

Includes bibliographical references and index.

1. Health Facilities—Administration. 2. Health
services administration. 3. Health facilities—United
States—Administration. I. Title [DNLM: 1. Health
services—Organization and administration. W 841
G624h]
RA971.G57   362.1'068   80-25645
ISBN: 0-89443-336-9

Library of Congress Catalog Card Number: 80-25645
ISBN: 0-89443-336-9

Printed in the United States of America

1 2 3 4 5

In Memoriam
I.A.G.

Table of Contents

Preface

As I reread and edited the manuscript for what appeared to be the hundredth time, I wondered if the potential readers of this volume—health services administrators, hospital administrators, managers in other health programs, health planners, and, last but hardly least, students in health administration programs—would understand my motivation in writing this book. Lest there be any confusion, I offer an explanation: my desire was to provide the reader with a broad background in the problems and issues involved in managing health services organizations. Each chapter is an attempt to analyze and interpret complex subjects and relate the analysis and interpretation to the "real world" of health administration.

Many of the areas of concern in this book have been subjected to such extensive research and writing that library shelves can be filled with works on these subjects; for example, scores of books have been written on motivation or strategic planning. I did not intend to provide summaries or literature reviews, and thus the reader in pursuit of a greater depth of knowledge must go beyond this text.

Like all writers, I am limited by my own knowledge and experience. In reviewing this text, I again realized how much of my experience (as a practicing administrator and consultant) is hospital-related. To those disinterested in hospitals, I suggest that the issues and experiences can be translated. To those who would like more cases from public health agencies or other organizations, I must simply acknowledge that present limitation. For all readers, whether administrators or students, I hope that the examples and cases, all of which are based on actual organizations, will be a useful starting point for analysis and discussion.

Finally, it was my wish to write a thoughtful and provocative book—I hope that goal has been achieved.

Seth B. Goldsmith
Amherst and
Northampton, Mass.
June, 1980

Acknowledgments

Acknowledgments are difficult for me to write, since I always have trouble knowing where to begin and end. Clearly, I owe a debt of gratitude to my colleagues Bob Gage and Juan Prawda, who prepared sections of this text. A debt is also owed to colleagues Lowell E. Bellin and Montague Brown, who reviewed the manuscript and offered helpful suggestions. Mike Brown at Aspen also deserves thanks for his encouragement and patience. Finally, a special note of appreciation to Sandra, Jonas, and Benjamin for their forbearance during the time I wrote this manuscript—"thanks for the space."

Chapter 1

Health Care Organizations and Their Environments

Environmental factors have a direct impact on health care organizations. The term *environmental factors* refers to those developments that occur external to the operations of a health care organization and over which the organization has essentially little control. Perhaps the most dramatic example is the cost of fuel oil. Prior to the Arab-Israeli War of October, 1973, and the subsequent oil embargoes and price hikes, the cost per gallon of the #6 crude oil that was used in a typical hospital was approximately 17 cents per gallon. By 1974, it was over 35 cents per gallon. Just between 1973 and 1974 the cost rose 58 percent. Translated into practical terms, a 300-bed hospital in New England that utilized 350,000 gallons per year was paying in 1974 almost 10 cents per gallon more than in 1973 and thus had an unanticipated fuel bill of an extra $35,000 for the year.

As a beginning for the analysis of the environment, four major groupings of factors that at one time or another affect or are likely to affect health care organizations can be identified: (1) demographic changes, (2) technological developments, (3) political changes, and (4) economic changes.

DEMOGRAPHIC CHANGES

Virtually every health care organization is affected by changes in any one of thousands of population shifts. Data from the National Health Interview Survey, conducted continuously by the National Center for Health Statistics, indicate that health care utilization varies by age, income, and geographical location, to mention just a few of the key variables. For example, families with incomes under $3,000 make more physician visits per year than families in other categories, 6.4 visits for the lowest income families contrasted with an average for all families of 5.1.[1] This simple statistic of physician visits per year also shows that whites tend to make more visits per year than blacks (5.1 compared with 4.7); people in the western states visit the physician more frequently than those in the north central states (5.9 compared with 4.7); and, as most people would predict, older people visit the physician more often than others in the population (6.5 visits per year for those over 65 compared with a national average for all ages of 5.1).[2]

Even when it comes to routine preventive care, important differences can be seen in different segments of the population. Illustrative of these differences are some of the following statements:

- 9 percent of the white population have never had a routine physical, while 15 percent of the nonwhite population have never had a routine physical.

- 73 percent of those with family incomes under $3,000 have had a physical, while 92 percent with incomes over $15,000 have had a routine physical examination.

- 55 percent of whites have been tested for glaucoma, while only 41 percent of nonwhites have had the test.

- 89 percent of whites and 80 percent of nonwhites have had their eyes examined.

- In women aged 45-64, 75 percent of white women have had a breast examination and Pap smear, while only 58 percent of nonwhite women have had a similar examination.[3]

In terms of hospital utilization, the average length of stay for persons 65 years and older is 11.9 days, while the average length of stay for the other age groups is 5.2 for those under 17 years of age, 5.1 for the 17-24 age group, 6.0 for the 25-34 age group, 6.9 for the 35-44 age group, and 9.2 for the 45-64 age group.[4] This information, together with the knowledge that the average life expectancy has increased by 3 years since 1960 and by almost 26 years (more than 50 percent) since 1910, makes it clear that a future health system will in part be shaped by factors outside its control (although admittedly life expectancy is perhaps one of the few factors over which the health system does exert some control). Thus, a more (or less) affluent country, changes in the racial or ethnic composition of the population, or a population that simply lives longer will all influence the shape of health systems.

Other demographic factors that directly affect the health system include population growth, shifts in residential patterns, and mobility. For example, between 1960 and 1977, births and migration added 36 million people to the U.S. population. These Americans annually generate an additional 184 million physician visits, 44 million community hospital patient days,[5] and thus a significant portion of the multi-billion dollar health bill.

As the U.S. population has grown, other things have occurred, most notably a shift out of what has been labeled the "industrial" Northeast to the sunbelt and from the urban centers to the suburbs. Why have states like Massachusetts seen population growths of almost half the national average, while California, Arizona, Florida, and other states have increased their populations by three, four, or five times the national average? Weather, jobs, and life style are clearly a large part of the answer—surely, it is not the availability or accessibility of high quality medical care!

Mobility of the population has also had an impact on the health system. For example, data from the U.S. census indicate that about 34 percent of the population had moved between 1975 and 1978; more than half of these moves involved significant shifts, that is, shifts between standard metropolitan statistical areas.[6] No doubt many of these moves also necessitated the establishment of new relationships with medical practitioners, a matter not always easily handled. While empirical work is generally lacking in this area, many persons have been met with disinterest and even disdain when they call a physician for the purpose of establishing a "relationship." A different type of example concerns the difficulty of making appropriate clinical connections and a latent fear, certainly based on some reality, that an unknown patient is likely to be "ping-ponged," that is, sent all over town for consultations and workups. One popular way of dealing with these concerns is to utilize the hospital emergency room as the major source of primary care—a clearly documented and costly alternative to seeing a primary care practitioner.

TECHNOLOGICAL DEVELOPMENTS

Computerized axial tomography (CAT) scanners, lasers, computers, and thousands of other technological "space age" developments, most of which were not initially conceived for the health field, have had a profound impact on health care.

The CAT scanner is certainly one of the most talked about technological innovations of the late 1970s. An advertisement for a scanner that appeared in the fall of 1978 notes that it "is the only CAT system presently available that can routinely perform high quality scans in 1 second. It's our response to the timely need of the medical community for fast and accurate diagnostic equipment." Other advertisements inform potential purchasers that a scanner can be purchased for under $100,000 or rented in mobile vans that can be set up in parking lots. When the scanners made their entrance into the medical marketplace in the mid-1970s, the prices were in the range of $650,000 and the scans took up to one minute.

The scanner itself is a device that passes an electronic beam through the body and then, by means of computers, regathers the images and presents them as a visual image of the body in much the same way that an x-ray does. For the patient, procedures that were often time-consuming, expensive, and painful have been eliminated by this fast new "machine."

Ultrasonography is another relatively new diagnostic "machine" that effectively maps the organs of the body. Sound waves are bounced off the organs and then processed through a computer so that the organs can be visualized on a screen. The value of this procedure can be demonstrated in amniocentesis, a procedure where amniotic fluid is extracted from the uterus for analysis of possible birth defects in a fetus. Without ultrasonography, determining the exact position of the fetus is a problem; without such a determination, a risk of accidentally puncturing the fetus is introduced. Prior to ultrasonography the physician would attempt to judge the fetus' position by "feel." Although this judgment was usually accurate, replacing it with a technologically advanced device is likely to cut down the errors to almost zero. Of course, a series of new problems may arise from such technological developments. To an extent, the National Institute for Health Technology is addressing some of these issues: for example, are CAT scanners or ultrasonography being overutilized to the detriment of the patient?

In the area of surgery, new developments in microsurgery have made it possible to rejoin severed limbs; laser knives can be utilized, thus shortening the length of time for surgery and reducing the risk from bleeding. New anesthetics have considerably lessened the risk of anesthesiology and to an extent opened up new patient populations, such as the very young and the very old, to the possibility of surgery. Because of advances through blood research, the life of many hemophiliacs has become considerably more bearable (and prolonged) than it had been just a generation ago.

A list of major technological developments could go on for pages, but the key point to remember is that these developments are often a result of technological changes that have occurred outside of the health care field. Many of these developments are intimately related to the development of the computer or to military needs. As *The New York Times* pointed out in its cover story of August 5, 1979,

> The Korean and VietNam wars both played a part in creating the new technology. Experimental physicists and mathematicians first employed to develop deadly new electronic gadgets for warfare (such as improved radar to track enemy missiles or infrared sensors to spot troop movements through nighttime jungles) began to look around for other areas in which to practice their skills.

POLITICAL CHANGES

Although many health professionals would like to consider themselves and their activities apolitical, in fact a great deal of what occurs in health care results from political decisions. For example, during the wage and price freeze of World War II, the Supreme Court declared that employee benefits, in particular health benefits, were a legitimate part of labor management bargaining and excluded such benefits from the wage and price freeze. This set the stage for the major escalation in third party health insurance coverage in the United States. At a different level, congressional action to exclude health care facilities from collective bargaining under the original Taft-Hartley legislation effectively kept wages and benefits in the health industry somewhat below those in the rest of the marketplace. A subsequent decision to extend collective bargaining rights to health care workers set the stage for a massive increase in the number of unionized health care workers.

Political decisions have been very much in the forefront of events concerning malpractice. Some states have effectively limited patients' ability to sue and collect from physicians by limiting liability or, in some instances, setting up state-dominated review and compensation panels. The states' intervention is a political act as a result of pressure generated by various special interest groups, in particular physicians.

Two final examples of how the political system affects health care involve abortions and health care costs. The key abortion decision was made on July 22, 1973, in the case of *Roe v. Wade*.[7] In this case, the U.S. Supreme Court ruled that all state statutes that prohibited abortions during the first trimester were unconstitutional. In a related case, *Doe v. Bolton*,[8] the Court ruled that two Georgia statutes, one requiring that those desiring abortions establish residency and one requiring that abortions be performed in hospitals approved by the Joint Commission on the Accreditation of Hospitals (JCAH), were unconstitutional. The practical implications of this ruling were that hospitals had to deal with the issue of whether and to what extent they were willing to offer abortion services. Some hospitals, such as one major New York teaching hospital, agreed to offer the service but then procrastinated for a year and a half and eventually decided to offer it on an inpatient basis only.

Because of the Supreme Court rulings, a new Catholic hospital in Massachusetts decided to avoid the entire problem and simply eliminate obstetric and related services. Recently, in Greenfield, Massachusetts, a merger between The Franklin County Public Hospital and the Farren Memorial Hospital, the latter being under Catholic auspices, was canceled over the issue of abortion, even though it had been agreed by virtually everyone involved, including the Health Systems Agency (HSA), that a merger was in the best interests of both institutions and the community. However, the issue of abortion is so controversial and has such profound implications for all concerned that it alone scuttled the proposal.

A more recent (July 2, 1979) decision of the Supreme Court in *Bellotti v. Baird* found that the Massachusetts statute that required unmarried minors to have their parents' consent for an abortion was unconstitutional.[9] Not only will such a finding change how minors are treated in terms of abortion consent, but also their consent for other medical procedures may now come under review.

A final example of the interaction between politics and the health system is the effort of various groups in Massachusetts to cut off medical reimbursement for abortions. If such a cutoff takes place, hospitals and other health care providers will be forced to make a difficult choice. They can either subsidize a needed and legal service, or they can deny welfare recipients the service and potentially face liability for this denial. Such a situation is very disconcerting to organizations that like to view themselves as both independent and stable. One response to dealing with these legal and regulatory issues has been the appointment of staff counsel in hospitals and other health care organizations.

Health Care Costs

In the area of health costs, the political system, particularly at a national level, has used its leverage to criticize the health system directly, blaming it in large part for the problems of the economy and looking for solutions that come together under the heading of regulating the health system. Thus, such measures as health planning, utilizations review, Professional Standards Review Organizations (PSROs), and HSAs are quite similar in that they are all political responses to problems in both our health system and our social system. Each one of these developments has an impact on the health system, and each is translated into new or different programs, changes in staff composition and numbers, and, ultimately, dollars.

The solutions envisioned by politicians have included cutting into the industry's, in particular hospitals', appetites for capital plants and equipment and increased fees. It is often suggested that some hospitals be closed. Quite clearly, a closed hospital would save health care dollars, but it would simultaneously present the political problems of unemployed hospital workers.

Finally, there is the issue of National Health Insurance, a political program that has been debated for half a century. Regardless of which plan is adopted, it will obviously cost more money and is likely to satisfy only a segment of the voting public. It should be recognized that the adoption of a National Health Insurance program is a political decision that will have a profound impact on each provider's community. While one cannot deny the influence providers have on such legislation, it must also be recognized that the political system will determine when it is in its own best interests (not necessarily the health system's) to implement such a program.

ECONOMIC CHANGES

To a great extent, the U.S. health system reflects the country's total economic system and is indeed very much affected by changes in that system.

On the supply side of the equation, the health system as it presently exists has thousands of large and relatively sophisticated suppliers (hospitals or large group practices) who in many instances have made the most expensive and extensive capital investments. In addition, there are hundreds of thousands of small professional suppliers, such as physicians, dentists, chiropractors, and podiatrists, each of whom may essentially operate independently; these small suppliers often have capital equipment that is not fully utilized, although it functions effectively as a convenience for the demander and supplier at a somewhat higher cost. For example, chiropractors often have extensive radiological equipment for diagnostic purposes because their relations with the community hospital and its radiologists are such that they are excluded from utilizing that service. [10,11] It should be noted here that, despite the competitive ethic in American society, particularly "business," it is extremely difficult for anyone or any group to enter into the "big business" of health care, both because of the capital investment requirement and because of social barriers. Indeed, only recently have the large proprietary hospitals and nursing homes, which tend to be financed by large corporations, been able to grow. Finally, society has set up enormous social and economic barriers to entry into the health care supply professions. Thus, a physician "supplier" is required to have an extended educational experience that is demanding both intellectually and economically. To ensure control of the various level supplies, a network of certification, licensure, and regulations has developed, all of which are justified on the basis of protecting society's best interests—usually clinical, not economic.

The demand side of the equation is complicated by consumers who enter a marketplace in differing ways, depending on their knowledge, attitudes, socio-economic status, or certain demographic factors. Further, once in the marketplace, they are not in a very strong position to know what they really need or the value of a given treatment. Thus, in most instances, they must trust the judgment of the providers.

Despite this oligarchic situation, there is a certain competition among providers. At different levels, providers are searching for a competitive edge over their perceived rivals. For example, in a small Maine community, two hospitals had been meeting about recruiting a neurosurgeon who would be on the staff of both hospitals. Certain types of cases would be restricted to one institution; other types of cases, to the other. This sharing, it was reasoned, would lower the capital investment in operating room equipment and supplies for each institution. After meetings had been proceeding for several months, the director of one hospital opened the morning newspaper and found a picture of the other hospital's director shaking hands with the newly appointed neurosurgeon and announcing that all neurosurgical operations would be performed at their hospital. No mention was made of the crosstown institution; in response to an inquiry, the now neurosurgeonless hospital was told that its "rival" had changed its mind. A postscript to this story is that 15 years later these two hospitals merged.

Competition for CAT scanners and open heart surgical rooms also produce popular stories. In the mid-1970s I served on a committee of the Columbia College of Physicians and Surgeons and The Presbyterian Hospital that was working on affiliation agreements with community hospitals for primary care residency training. Our major function was to meet with medical and administrative staffs of community hospitals in order to ascertain their interest in becoming affiliated with Columbia and Presbyterian. At one such meeting at a hospital in northern New Jersey, a physician in the community hospital asked us very bluntly if an affiliation meant that Presbyterian would get the CAT scanner. Although no one could say authoritatively what would happen in such a situation, we did respond that it was a distinct possibility. At that point, the physician who had asked the question and happened to be a former president of the medical staff suggested adjourning our meeting.

A different dimension of how the health system reflects the total economic system is that of specialization. From most perspectives, the United States has a specialized economy that finds its ultimate manifestation in the automobile assembly plant. The health system, which is or should be part of the larger social system, has become through design and/or neglect a very separate system from the rest of social or human services. Thus, it is often called the "non-health system." But, in fact, the non-health system is one small part of the larger nonsystems, i.e., the fragmentation and specialization within the total economic system.

Government economic policies affect the health system dramatically. For example, a welfare policy such as the "War on Poverty" provides resources for the health system. Because of the interest on that front during the Johnson presidency, neighborhood health centers and, to some extent, other community-based programs were developed. Some of these programs, such as Medicaid for the poor or Medicare for the elderly, actually enfranchised patients through fiscal mechanisms. In economic terms, these programs shifted the demand curve outward by bringing new buyers into the market. Since the system did not have a great deal of excess capacity, they also necessitated alternative arrangements to meet demand. Thus, in certain areas of New York and other large metropolitan areas, neighborhood Medicaid clinics were established to fulfill the needs of Medicaid recipients. In a sense, the health system responded by utilizing the Willie Sutton principle, "going to where the money is." Some observers of the health system believe that government economic policy will eventually doom the government hospitals, since the newly enfranchised patients will vote with their dollars and use their Medicaid cards in a more attractive voluntary hospital. Clearly, despite financial enfranchisement, patterns of care change slowly—witness the Duke

Medical Center, where the Medicaid card holders still sit on hard chairs waiting for house staff while the private patients sit on cushioned chairs awaiting the professors.[12]

The health system must also respond to the demands of the general economy by facing the costs of inflation. For example, in the past several years, inflation has driven the costs of construction up by approximately 12 percent per year. A health facility being built, renovated, or expanded is certainly not immune to those costs and, like most prudent investors, tries to minimize future expenses via mechanisms such as building shell space. Thus, institutions that seem to be overexpanding are in fact simply hedging their bets against an uncertain but likely more expensive future.

Energy is perhaps the best example of the health system as a victim. A group practice, neighborhood health center, or hospital must purchase gas, oil, or electricity in the same manner as any other organization. Other examples of dramatic increases in essentially uncontrollable expenses for institutions include

- food, which increased 17.9 percent from 1972 to 1973 and another 14.6 percent between 1973 and 1974

- interest on working capital, which increased 49.7 percent between 1973 and 1974

- electricity, which increased 18.3 percent between 1973 and 1974

- rubber and miscellaneous plastics, which increased 21.1 percent between 1973 and 1974

These skyrocketing costs have obviously affected health care institutions—but unlike most commercial or industrial concerns, they cannot easily pass on these additional costs. The mechanisms for rate increases vary from state to state; but, in general, there is a time lag, and the ability of the organization to make up its losses is limited.

Work stoppages or failures, as well as new union agreements in other industries, also affect the health industry, since it is a major purchaser of many products and services. Consider the implications of a failure at Chrysler: 120,000 unemployed people and their families with limited financial access to health services—clearly, a catastrophe for all systems in the United States!

Another side of the coin for the health system is the impact of the oil crisis on driving habits. With the speed limit reduction the number of traffic deaths has been cut from 56,000 in 1972 to 47,000 in 1977. This, too, translates into different demands and usage patterns for the health system. It has been argued in some quarters that the major causes of death in the United States—heart disease, cancer, and stroke—are very heavily related to our economic system. For example, the elimination of smoking could have significant salubrious effects on the health of the population, but it certainly would not have a positive effect on the economic health of the tobacco industry. Indeed, the ouster of former secretary of Health, Education and Welfare, Joseph Califano, was in part attributed to his aggressive stand against the tobacco industry in the interest of the public's health.

Perhaps no example is more timely than that of the conflict between the nuclear industry and health. Energy, particularly cheap energy, has become so important in our society that, despite seemingly obvious health risks and a good deal of uncertainty (in all fairness, there are also benefits, but they are most often presented by the nuclear industry), nuclear power plant expansion has continued.

In sum, then, the health industry is both a party to the nation's economic developments and the recipient of its benefits and problems. The health industry itself has not and is not likely ever to be in a position in which it can be said that "what's good for the health industry is good for America;" but it appears that the time is near when it can be said that what is bad for the health industry is certainly not very good for America. Perhaps illustrative of this point is the fact that there is more "health care" in the cost of a Chevrolet than in the cost of steel.

CASE STUDY

The Metroplex Eye, Ear, and Throat Hospital

The free-standing specialty eye, ear, nose, and throat hospital appears to be an endangered species. In 1955, there were 51 such hospitals in the United States, with a total complement of 2,486 beds and an average daily census of 1,446 patients (58.1 percent occupancy). Such hospitals were found in virtually every large city. In general, those hospitals could be categorized into two groups: (1) small (under 50 beds) proprietary facilities and (2) larger, not-for-profit institutions, nine of which had over 100 beds.

In 1975, there were only 20 independent eye, ear, nose, and throat hospitals remaining, including the several that had been opened in the intervening 20-year period. These hospitals had a complement of 1,463 beds (a decline of 41 percent in the total since 1955) and an average daily census of 930 (a 36 percent decline). Because the decline in bed complement exceeded the decline in patients, total occupancy rate increased to 63.5 percent, still extremely low by comparison with general hospitals, where the national mean in recent years has hovered just short of 75 percent. In the same 1955-1975 period, the number of all short-term nonfederal hospitals increased from 5,237 to 5,979, an increase of 14 percent, while the total number of beds in such hospitals increased almost 25 percent, from 568,000 to 708,000.

Among the cities losing their speciality eye, ear, nose, and throat hospitals were Chicago, Baltimore, and Washington, D.C. (Table 1-1). In the greater New York area, Bronx Eye and Ear Infirmary, Brooklyn Eye and Ear, and Harlem Eye and Ear all closed within this period. The indisputable conclusion must, therefore, be that specialty eye and ear hospitals have not fared well in recent years, even though the environment for hospitals in general has, until recently, been relatively benign—indeed, even supportive of the kinds of services offered to the clients of such institutions.

Since 1902, the Metroplex Eye, Ear, and Throat Hospital has been successfully operated as an institution whose name is synonymous with high quality medical care. Its basic operating statistics have been

- hospital size: 191 beds

- occupancy rate: 69%

- average length of stay: 4.4 days

(Table 1-2 furnishes some service statistics.) Its staff has always included individuals with national and international reputations, it is fiscally viable (having one of the lowest per diem charges in the region), and its occupancy rate is within a reasonable range for its type of hospital (Table 1-3). From the hospital's perspective, its main problems are (1) an old physical plant that is in violation of many sections of the life safety code, (2) an inability to arrange an affiliation or "merge" agreement that allows it to maintain its independence, and (3) the desire of the HSA to close the hospital.

On October 17, 1975, the following story appeared on the second page of the *Metroplex Gazette:*

METROPLEX EYE, EAR, AND THROAT HOSPITAL TO BE CLOSED AS FIRE TRAP

It was announced today that the Metroplex Eye, Ear, and Throat Hospital would not be granted an approval for its $20 million project renovation by the Metroplex Health Systems Agency. Ms. Jennifer Greene, executive director of the agency, said during a press conference that "Metro's days are numbered; it is in violation of so many sections of the life safety code that it is really a fire trap."

Responding to these charges, Hiram Walker, the hospital's administrator since 1946, said that the hospital was "sound as a dollar and that the violations were minor," and he also declared that "Metro has the highest weekday occupancy rate in the city and the lowest per diem charges." He also stated that Metro was a critical facility in the region and that a suit against the Health Systems Agency was contemplated.

Table 1-1 Single Speciality Eye, Ear, Nose, and Throat Hospitals Closed Since 1955

	Hospital	Year Established	Status For Profit?	Location	Bed Size	1955 (%) Occupancy
1	Los Angeles Eye & Ear	1925	Yes	Los Angeles, CA	21	42.8
2	Green's Eye	1928	No	San Francisco, CA	35	25.7
3	Page & Fowler Private	1946	Yes	Orlando, FL	10	N.R.
4	Episcopal Eye, Ear & Throat	1897	No	Washington, DC	100	54.0
5	Griffy Eye & Ear Infirmary	1938	Yes	Robinson, IL	6	16.6
6	Kuhn Clinic	1941	Yes	Hammond, IN	12	33.0
7	Citizens	1934	Yes	Anderson, IN	15	N.R.
8	Illinois Eye & Ear Inf.	1858	No	Chicago, IL	134	53.7
9	Baltimore Eye, Ear & Throat Charity	1815	No	Baltimore, MD	68	86.7
10	Presbyterian Eye, Ear & Throat	1876	No	Baltimore, MD	40	25.0
11	Wolfson Nose & Throat	1944	Yes	Boston, MA	8	12.5
12	Barnett Hospital & Clinic	1923	No	Detroit, MI	15	.06
13	Missouri Trachoma	1925	No	Rolla, MO	65	53.8
14	Casebeer Eye, Ear, Nose & Throat	1940	Yes	Butte, MT		44
15	Newark Eye & Ear Inf.	1880	No	Newark, NJ	65	60
16	Endamal	1945	Yes	New York, NY	27	N.R.
17	Brooklyn Eye & Ear	1868	No	Brooklyn, NY	137	—
18	Harlem Eye & Ear	1881	No	New York, NY	48	N.R.
19	Bronx Eye & Ear	1903	No	Bronx, NY	58	59.8
20	Buffalo Eye & Ear	1876	No	Buffalo, NY	14	64.2
21	Sahor EENT	1904	Yes	Columbus, OH	6	50
22	Gemmill	1936	Yes	Monaca, PA	17	35.2
23	McGogh Private	1946	Yes	Trafford, PA	9	55.5

24 Hooks-English	1926	Yes	Bristol, TN	10	30
25 Isbell Eye	1948	Yes	Chattanooga, TN	26	11.5
26 Jones EENT	1923	Yes	Johnson City, TN	25	32.0
27 McKee-Wilson	1945	Yes	Johnson City, TN	31	58.0
28 Christenberry Infirmary	1920	Yes	Knoxville, TN	12	N.R.
29 Woodward	1941	Yes	Arlington, TX	10	N.R.
30 Wilkinson	1949	Yes	Dallas, TX	6	33.3
31 Strickland ENT	1948	Yes	Greenville, TX	5	20.0
32 Houston ENT	1927	No	Houston, TX	23	56.2
33 Hurst ENT	1918	No	Longnew, TX	25	—
34 Harper ENT	1951	Yes	Port Arthur, TX	8	—
35 Adams	1947	Yes	Wichita Falls, TX	7	N.R.

Table 1-2 Service Statistics for 1965, 1970, and 1975

	1965	1970	1975
Outpatient visits			
Eye Service	51,110	47,019	52,874
ENT & Plastic	44,731	46,111	47,310
Inpatient admissions			
Eye	4,014	4,117	4,397
ENT	5,297	5,101	4,897
Plastic	931	1,066	1,251
Surgical procedures			
Eye	3,719	4,303	5,001
ENT	4,881	4,462	4,509
Plastic	714	909	1,302

Table 1-3 Comparative Staffing Ratios of Eye and Ear Hospitals

	Metroplex	Massachusetts Eye and Ear	Wills/ Philadelphia	Pittsburgh Eye andEar
Number of Beds	191	174	120	172
Number of Staff	483	818	440	425
Staff/Bed Ratio	2.52	4.70	3.66	2.47
Occupancy (%)	69.0	83.3	72.5	75.0

Discussion Questions

1. What external factors are likely to have played a part in the hospital's problems?
2. How can these factors be researched and validated?
3. Who should be responsible for environmental scanning? Board, medical staff, administrators, or department heads?
4. What system can be developed for environmental scanning in a health services organization?
5. What should be Metroplex's strategy for dealing with its future?

NOTES

1. National Center for Health Statistics, *Physician Visits, Volume and Interval Since Last Visit, United States—1975,* PHS Pub. No. 79-1556, April, 1979, p. 21.

2. Ibid., pp. 19, 22.

3. National Center for Health Statistics, *Use of Selected Medical Procedures Associated with Preventive Care, United States—1973,* HRA Pub. No. 77-1538, March, 1977.

4. National Center for Health Statistics, *Current Estimates from the Health Interview Survey, United States—1978,* PHS Pub. No. 80-1551, November, 1979.

5. Hospital bed data estimate is based on 1977 data from American Hospital Association that indicates 1,215 patient days per 1,000 for community hospitals.

6. U.S. Bureau of the Census, *Statistical Abstract of the United States: 1979,* 100th ed., 1979, p. 40.

7. *Roe v. Wade,* 410 U.S. 113 (1973).

8. *Doe v. Bolton,* 410 U.S. 179, 198 (1973).

9. *Bellotti v. Baird,* U.S., 61 L. Ed. 2d 797, 99 S. Ct. Rep 3035 (July 2, 1979).

10. G. Silver, "Chiropractic: Professional Controversy and Public Policy," *American Journal of Public Health* 70 (1980): 348-350.

11. C.E. Yesalis et al., "Does Chiropractic Utilization Substitute for Less Available Medical Services?" *American Journal of Public Health* 70 (1980): 415-417.

12. S.B. Thacher et al., "Primary Health Care in an Academic Medical Center," *American Journal of Public Health* 68 (1978): 853-857.

Chapter 2

An Overview of the U.S. Health System

A basic question managers must ask is, What is the nature of the system being managed? For most people, the health system means utilization, an occasional visit to a physician (i.e., four or five visits per year) or an occasional and usually short stay in a health care institution. To a manager, however, the health system can be analyzed in a variety of ways: in terms of expenditures, facilities, manpower, and patients (or clients, consumers, or users).

HEALTH EXPENDITURES

In the calendar year 1978, the expenditures for health care totaled $192 billion, or $863 per capita. This enormous amount of money represented 9.1 percent of the gross national product.[1] How were these $192 billion spent? By whom? For what? With what controls?

Most of the dollars (approximately 87 percent for the past decade) have been spent on personal health services. The bulk of these personal health dollars pay for hospital services, while other significant percentages are for physician services, nursing home care, drugs, and dental services. The nonpersonal health service expenditures are categorized as those associated with government public health activities, with prepayment and administration, and with research and medical facilities construction.

Hospitals consume by far the lion's share of the health dollars, but this has not always been the case. Prior to 1939, physician services were the largest single area of health care expenditures, followed closely by hospital services. Subsequent to World War II and up to the present time, hospital expenses have exceeded all other items by a significant degree. In the period of 1928-1929, hospital care represented 18 percent of the total health expenditures. By 1939-1940, these expenditures represented 25 percent; by the pre-Medicare/Medicaid period of 1964-1965, this percentage had grown to almost 34 percent; and by 1978, the total had reached almost 40 percent. During this same period, expenditures for physician services had gone from 28 percent in the 1928-1929 time period, to 25 percent in the 1939-1940 period, to 34 percent in 1964-1965; by 1978, physician services, although over $432 billion (or over nine times the entire health expenditure in 1929), represented less than 20 percent of the total health expenditures.[2]

What had occurred? Why have health expenditures escalated so dramatically, and why have the shifts in expenditure patterns been so great? Several explanations have been offered, including population growth, inflation, the cost of technology, and financing patterns.

Some of the dramatic increases in health expenditures are explained simply by the fact that there are considerably more Americans today than there were 10, 20, or 30 years ago. More people demand more services, and older people—who are increasing in number because of a longer life expectancy—also demand more services.

Inflation is a second major factor in the trend toward increased expenditures. How much of the increase can be explained by inflation is debatable, but it is clear that a 1950 dollar is not the equivalent of a present dollar and that most bills must be paid in present value currency. In one examination of the reasons for the increase in health expenditures, it was found that inflation accounted for 44 percent of the increase in health expenditures between 1950 and 1965 and 43 percent of the increased expenditures between 1971 and 1974.[3] A different report indicated that "52 percent of the $38.4 billion increase from fiscal year 1965 to fiscal year 1972 reflected a rise in prices." In explaining the remaining rise, this article noted that "10 percent ($3.8 billion) was the result of population growth, and the remaining 38 percent ($14.7 billion) was attributable to greater utilization of services and the introduction of new medical techniques."[4]

Another way of looking at these increases is to examine "input factors." In a 1978 review of the increases in hospital spending between 1970 and 1977, Gibson and Fisher found that

> Approximately 34 percent of this 1970-1977 increase reflected higher wages and salaries for a 1970 level of employees, and 23 percent resulted from the price of goods and services that hospitals had to purchase to maintain a 1970 level of services. The remaining 42 percent resulted from changes in the resources applied to a day of care. These resource changes, sometimes referred to as "intensity" changes, include the utilization of greater numbers of employees and/or more highly skilled employees, increased use of services (laboratory tests, X-rays, etc.) per day of care, and the provision of new and more expensive kinds of services such as computerized tomographic scans or heart bypass surgery.[5]

Not only has the use of the health care dollar changed, but also the source of the revenue has shifted. This shift has had and will continue to have a profound effect on management of health care organizations. The two most important shifts are related to the payer and the source of the revenue. In terms of the payer, direct patient payments have decreased from 88.5 percent prior to 1929 to 30 percent in the fiscal 1977 period. During that same period, third party payments have increased up to 70 percent, of which 27.6 percent comes from private health insurance, 2.0 percent from philanthropy, and 40 percent from government. Indeed, Medicaid and Medicare, which did not come into existence until the mid-1960s, account for 21 percent of all personal health expenditures. Government now not only pays 40 percent of the total health bill, but it also pays 55 percent of the hospital bill and 24 percent of the physician's bill.

Along with these increased payments from the government has come an increased control of the expenditures. For example, virtually every major health bill that has passed through Congress since the late 1960s has been supported on the basis that it would contain or reduce health care costs. Kinzer, however, of the Massachusetts Hospital Association, argues that "regulation is now costing Massachusetts hospitals between $60 million and $80 million a year, but this does not even count capital costs that result."[6] At the institution level, Kinzer found that a 471-bed hospital "reported that regulations were costing it $354,000 a year with the heaviest part of that in accounting, where added costs are $134,500 a year."[7] Overall, the institution calculated that regulations were costing $2.22 per patient day.

The general perspective of most institutional and individual providers is that the government regulates too much and rather arbitrarily. One California family practitioner notes that "in 1967 under the state's Medi-Cal physicians in my own county of San Bernardino were generally receiving $6 for a regular follow-up office visit. Today [1977] for the same office visit they get a maximum of $8.38 from the Medi-Cal while the average charge to the private patient is roughly $14."[8] Government, he and others argue, tends to cut or freeze payments arbitrarily in order to meet its own operating deficits and thus encourages unsatisfactory forms of delivering care, such as "Medicaid mills." They argue that these mills exist simply because of the economic constraints imposed on the practitioners.

Despite these massive expenditures, there is clearly a lack of equity in the U.S. health system. Many observers argue that this is inevitable, since our society is fundamentally inequitable and the health system is simply a reflection of that. It should be recognized, however, that some of this inequity is institutionalized, even by such government programs as Medicaid in which every state has considerable latitude in setting the levels of eligibility, the quantity, and to some extent the quality of services that will be available.

HOSPITALS

As noted earlier, hospitals take the lion's share of every pie in the health system except the profit. Hospitals are usually categorized by ownership—governmental, nongovernmental, or proprietary (for profit)—and type of services offered—general medical and surgical, specialty (ear, nose, throat), or category of patient (children's hospital). Hospitals are also categorized according to the length of stay in the institution: short-term, which means that more than 50 percent of the patients stayed less than 30 days, and long-term, which means that more than 50 percent stayed more than 30 days.

Since 1963, the number of hospitals in the United States has been fairly constant, although from 1953 through 1963 there was an increase of over 1,000 institutions. As of 1978, these 7,015 facilities had 1.4 million beds, which is five percent more beds than they had in 1950 when there were approximately 35 million fewer people in this country. During this same time period, the total number of admissions doubled for hospitals; the number of births increased from 2.7 million in 1950 to 4.2 million in 1960 and dropped to 3 million in 1974 and 3.2 million in 1978. Throughout this period the personnel per 100 census increased from 84 to more than 250 and the ambulatory visits to hospitals increased from 99 million in 1962 to 263 million in 1978.[9]

What is going on? What is behind all these numbers that at first glance do not seem to make any sense whatsoever! Fundamentally, what has occurred is an internal reorganization of bed utilization. Psychotropic drugs have allowed many persons to function outside of psychiatric hospitals so that the number of psychiatric beds has been decreased from 620,000 in 1950 to 285,000 in 1977. Other shifts in incidence and treatment of diseases have resulted in similar decreases, such as the decrease in the number of beds in tuberculosis and respiratory disease hospitals from 72,000 beds in 1950 to 3,315 in 1977. During these same 27 years, however, the number of short-term hospital beds has increased from 505,000 to 975,000, and the number of staff per 100 census has increased from 178 to 316.

The heart of the hospital system is the community hospital—the short-term, nonfederal hospital that provides a range of general medical and surgical services. In 1977 these 5,881 hospitals had a total of 969,000 beds. While there is clearly a great variety of hospitals, some basic data regarding the "average" community hospital can be identified. The mythical average hospital has a total of 165 beds and is located in a community where there is a 4.5 bed per 1,000 population ratio and where there are 169 physicians per 100,000 population. Incidentally, the average bed size of hospitals ranges from a low of 104 in the Mountain states to a high of 256 in the Middle Atlantic region; physician population ratios also show dramatic differences, ranging from 214 per 100,000 in New England to 117 in the East South Central region. The occupancy in the "typical American hospital" is

75 percent, with an average length of stay of 7.7 days and an annual inpatient turnover rate of 35.5 percent.

The average expense per inpatient day in 1977 was $174, of which approximately 60 percent was in personnel costs (salary/wages and benefits) for an employee who in 1977 averaged $10,082 per year. The 1977 assets of the institution, e.g., the physical plant, were calculated to be worth almost $63,000 per bed; however, to replace the physical facility would likely cost considerably more than $100,000 per bed.

In terms of the utilization of short-term hospitals, data gathered from the National Center for Health Statistics shows that there are considerable differences in hospitalization rates between men and women and different age groups. It was found that in 1978 there were 139 male and 192 female discharges per 1,000 population and that the length of stay varied only slightly between the sexes. In explaining this higher rate of discharge by sex, the authors note that "the number and rate of discharges are always higher for females than for males because of the large number of women in the child bearing ages (15-44 years) who are hospitalized for deliveries and other obstetrical conditions."[10]

AMBULATORY CARE

Ambulatory care is provided in a variety of locations: physicians' offices, hospital outpatient departments, hospital emergency rooms, and a range of other facilities.

Of the care in a physician's office, 60 percent occurs in the office of solo practitioners, while the remaining care is delivered in some variant of a group setting. The largest percentage of visits are made to general or family practitioners (38.4 percent); 11.6 percent are made to internists, 10.3 percent to pediatricians, and 8.3 percent to obstetricians and gynecologists.[11] In addition to the 424,000 practicing physicians in the United States, of whom approximately 70 percent are in office-based practice, there is a variety of other health practitioners. Dentists provide over 332 million annual visits for patients, podiatrists 24 million visits, and chiropractors 90 million visits. [12, 13]

Recent preliminary data from the National Ambulatory Medical Care Survey indicate that on the average there are 2.8 office visits per year per person.[11] These data closely correspond to the information previously available from the National Center for Health Statistics, which indicated that there were approximately 4.9 physician visits per person per year, of which 69.6 percent or 3.4 physician visits per year per person were to office-based physicians. Although the number of physician visits per year has increased slightly per year, these increases appear to be related more closely to the collection methodology than to significant changes in consumer ambulatory use patterns.[14]

A different picture is seen in the outpatient clinics and emergency rooms of hospitals. For example, in 1964, hospitals reported a total of 125 million outpatient visits; a decade later the number had more than doubled. Further, this occurred at a time when the national population had increased by 20 percent, outpatient departments had become deficit operations, the number of physicians was increasing, and the number of hospitals with outpatient clinics was declining. Simultaneously, emergency department visits increased at an even greater rate. In 1964, there were 26 million emergency department visits; by 1974, the total had mushroomed to over 71 million visits. Perhaps of even greater significance are the various studies indicating that a majority of the emergency department patients are utilizing that facility for primary care.[15]

The five most common complaints of patients making office visits to physicians have been found to be (1) pain, swelling, injury of lower extremity (3.6 percent); (2) pain, swelling, injury to the back region (2.9 percent); (3) sore throat (2.8 percent); (4) pain, swelling, injury to the upper extremity (2.7 percent); and (5) abdominal pain (2.5 percent). The most common findings that have resulted from the range of office visits have been a need for medical or special examination (7.6 percent); a need for medical or surgical examination (5.0 percent); essential benign hypertension (4.0 percent); prenatal care (3.6 percent); and acute upper respiratory infection (3.2 percent). This has been translated into a history or examination in 69 percent of the visits, a blood pressure check in 33 percent of the visits, and/or a laboratory test in 23 percent of the visits. The most frequently offered therapeutic service has been the prescription of a drug (42.8 percent of the time), followed by medical counseling (13.6 percent of the time), and an injection (12.5 percent of the time). Almost 95 percent of the visits have lasted less than 30 minutes; 45 percent last less than 10 minutes, 26 percent between 11 and 15 minutes, and 20 percent between 16 and 30.[11]

Other ambulatory health care facilities that provide important services include the university-based student health centers, clinics sponsored by labor organizations, industrial clinics that can be found in plants and other places where large numbers of persons are employed, neighborhood health centers, free clinics, family planning clinics, and community mental health center programs.

OTHER HEALTH CARE INSTITUTIONS AND PROVIDERS

It is sometimes difficult to know the boundaries of the "health system." What should be included and excluded within a definition of health services, as opposed to other social services? For example, should the definition include pharmacies that not only dispense prescription drugs but also sell billions of dollars of nonprescription over-the-counter preparations that people use to self-medicate? Clearly, the "corner drugstore" for many is the source of "primary care;" thus, it is important to count it in a tally of health care resources. What about the range of nontraditional healers, such as herbalists and therapeutic masseurs? No doubt they help people. For the most part, however, they are excluded from the traditional health system in that they cannot utilize the system's major resources (such as hospitals), and they often have only limited access to its insurance mechanisms. For the purposes of this review, they shall generally be excluded. The extent of their involvement in the health system should be recognized, however. For example, in one report it was found that

> an estimated 3.6 percent of the population (7.5 million persons) used the services of a chiropractor; 2.4 percent (5.0 million persons) consulted a podiatrist or chiropodist; and 1.6 percent (3.2 million persons) used the services of a physical therapist.[16]

Unfortunately, it should be noted that the exclusion of some nontraditional healers, such as midwife and the chiropractor, is of a political nature and is based on the historical power of organized medicine. For example, the history of midwifery in the United States clearly demonstrates that the early twentieth century campaign of the organized medical professionals, in particular the professors of obstetrics in the major medical schools, against midwives in America was not based on sound scientific evidence but to a major extent on their self-interest. Indeed, had the United States followed the lead of England at that time, this country would have had a totally different type of obstetrical care—perhaps a different health system.

In addition to the range of mental health and specialized facilities such as schools for the mentally retarded, halfway houses, and schools and homes for people with physical handicaps, the nursing home has in the past two decades taken on great importance in the health system. These facilities now number over 23,000 and provide care at different levels to over 1 million people. As consumers of health care dollars, the nursing home industry has rapidly moved into a major category, accounting for 8.2 percent of the expenditures in 1978.

Managers manage not only physical resources, such as a building, or finances but also people. The 1978 estimates of the number of persons employed in health occupations were 4.6 million, of whom 70 percent (3.2 million) work in hospitals. The largest groups of these workers are registered nurses (1.1 million), nursing aides (also 1 million), and practical nurses (402,000). These three groups account for over 50 percent of all the health workers. Physicians and osteopaths number 424,000; pharmacists, 136,000; dentists, 117,000; clinical laboratory technical staff, 208,000; and radiology technicians, 97,000. It is interesting to note that, in the highest paid and most autonomous professional groups, males predominate; 89 percent of the physicians, 98 percent of the dentists, and 83 percent of the pharmacists are male. In nursing, females account for 97 percent of the registered nurses, 97 percent of the practical nurses, and 87 percent of the nursing aides. [9, 17, 18]

In 1977, there were 134 medical and osteopathic schools, graduating more than 15,000 physicians per year. Augmenting this physician supply were physicians trained in medical schools abroad. In 1977, over 7,000 of these graduates were admitted to the United States as immigrants, and 5,851 graduates of foreign medical schools were licensed to practice in the United States.[17] Despite the occasional cries of a physician shortage, the number of physicians per 100,000 population has steadily increased for almost two generations, and all targets for a physician population ratio have been exceeded. In 1977, there were 198 physicians per 100,000 population. The problem of uneven distribution has persisted, however. For example, Massachusetts has 241 physicians per 100,000, while Mississippi has 105 per 100,000. This type of discrepancy has tended to keep the states with good supplies of physicians at the high end of the scale, while those at the bottom end have also stayed in place. These statistics also mask discrepancies within a state, region, or even community. For example, in the western part of Massachusetts, there are towns with an ample, perhaps excessive, supply of physicians, while there are other communities with few or, in some cases, no physicians. Another problem with the statistics is that they reveal little about the distribution of physicians within specialties. For example, until recently, the number of family practitioners was quite low, while the number of radiologists and surgeons was unnecessarily high.

The 59 dental schools in the United States graduate approximately 5,900 dentists each year. The 1,352 nursing schools graduate 78,000 new nurses each year. It should be noted that the nursing schools include those within hospitals (the traditional three-year diploma schools), the two-year community college programs, and the four-year collegiate programs. Training for other health care occupations may range from the Ph.D. level for clinical laboratory work, to master's level for health administration, to baccalaureate level in many areas, and finally to on-the-job training for aide positions.

THE NEW ORGANIZATIONS IN TOWN

It sometimes appears that the past decade or two has spawned an entire generation of organizations whose prime concern is either regulating or redirecting the health system. Some of these organizations are not actually new but rather reincarnations of older and similarly oriented programs.

The regulators are likely to be on any manager's mind. In the health care field, there are literally hundreds of organizations involved in regulation; others want to be. For example, the Federal Trade Commission is interested in instigating some antitrust activity in the health field, and the Federal Communications Commission has expressed concern over the proliferation of sophisticated electronic medical equipment that is allegedly causing problems with certain communications equipment. At the federal level, in addition to the organizations fully involved with health, which include primarily large sections of the Department of Health and Human Services—most notably the Health Care Financing Administration—other non-health-related executive branch departments, such as the Bureau of the Budget, also play critical roles in the health system. The federal government also funds programs such as Health Systems Agencies or Professional Standards Review Organizations, which are quasi-governmental in nature and have a great impact upon local institutions and programs.

State governments have similar structures: health departments that often have considerable regulatory power and various related organizations, such as rate commissions and health planning departments.

At the local level, there is also a range of government or government-related health planning bodies and, again, some regulatory agencies, such as boards of health.

Organizations for personal professional development, special medical interest groups, and lobbying groups appear to be omnipresent. Virtually every health profession (or group of workers) has its own organization. Disease- or problem-oriented organizations are also in abundance, as are the lobbyists—some of which tend to focus on organizations, such as the American Medical Association or the American Hospital Association, and some on fund-raising for activities to combat specific diseases, such as alcoholism.

The picture is one of an expensive, complex, and quite fragmented system. Clearly, the health system is not simply a group of well-defined and integrated components that all relate to a common goal. On the contrary, it is a system with considerable overlap, waste, and a multiplicity of goals.

NOTES

1. Health Care Financing Administration, *Health Care Financing Trends* 1, no. 1 (Fall 1979): 3.

2. R.M. Gibson, "National Health Expenditures, 1978," *Health Care Financing Review* 1, no. 1 (Summer 1979): 23-24.

3. R.M. Gibson and M.S. Mueller, "National Health Expenditures, Fiscal Year, 1976," *Social Security Bulletin* 40, no. 4 (April 1977): 14.

4. B.S. Cooper and N.L. Worthington, "National Health Expenditures, 1929-1972," *Social Security Bulletin* 36, no. 1 (January 1973): 13.

5. R.M. Gibson and C.R. Fisher, "National Health Expenditures, Fiscal Year 1977," *Social Security Bulletin* 41, no. 7 (July 1978): 10-11.

6. D.M. Kinzer, *Health Controls Out of Control: Warnings to the Nation from Massachusetts* (Chicago: Teach'em, 1977), p. 73.

7. Ibid., p. 75.

8. N.P. Krikes, "Behind the Rise in Health Care Costs," testimony delivered before the California Subcommittee on Health and Welfare, Sacramento, CA, December 12, 1977.

9. American Hospital Association, *Hospital Statistics,* 1979 ed. (Chicago: American Hospital Association, 1979).

10. National Center for Health Statistics, *Utilization of Short Stay Hospitals, Annual Summary for the United States, 1978,* PHS Pub. No. 80-1797, March, 1980, p. 2.

11. National Center for Health Statistics, *The National Ambulatory Care Survey: 1976, Summary, Advanced Data,* No. 30, July 13, 1978.

12. American Medical Association, Center for Health Services Research and Development, *Profile of Medical Practice,* 1979, p. 154.

13. National Center for Health Statistics, *Health Resources Statistics* 1976-1977, PHS Pub. No. 79-1509, 1979.

14. National Center for Health Statistics, *Physician Visits, Volume and Interval Since Last Visit, United States—1971,* HRA Pub. No. 75-1524, March, 1975, pp. 28-30.

15. L.J. Taubenhaus, "The Non-Scheduled Patient in Emergency Department and Walk-In Clinic," *Bulletin of New York Academy of Medicine* 49, no. 5 (May 1973): 419-426.

16. National Center for Health Statistics, *Advance Data,* No. 24, March 24, 1978.

17. U.S. Bureau of the Census, *Statistical Abstract of the United States: 1979,* 100th ed., 1979, p. 108.

18. U.S. Department of Health, Education and Welfare, *A Study of the Participation of Women in the Health Care Industry Labor Force,* HRA Pub. No. 77-644, June, 1977.

Chapter 3

The Health Care Industry: A Managerial Model

Health care organizations can generally be classified into three basic groups, depending on their financial sponsorship: (1) for profit, (2) not for profit, or (3) governmental. This classification results in a significant number of anatomical and physiological differences which to a great extent affect the organization's management processes.

THE PROPRIETARY SECTOR

The first classification, for profit, includes the independent practices of physicians, dentists, and other providers. Often run as small businesses, some of these practices have become so sophisticated that they utilize a range of subcontractors for business and professional functions. At the most sophisticated end of the range of for-profit providers are large group practices, which are likely to be organized as partnerships, employ hundreds of professionals and nonprofessionals, and own real estate and a host of other business ventures (often under separate corporate entities).

Inpatient facilities are a more complex form of for-profit organizations. These facilities have in the past few years experienced remarkable growth, particularly in the areas of hospitals and nursing homes owned by large chains and publicly held corporations such as Hospital Corporation of America (HCA), Humana, or Holiday Inn. Some private single specialty hospitals, such as psychiatric hospitals, have managed to survive the past few decades. As was noted in Chapter 1, however, the proprietary ear, nose, and throat hospitals have not fared well during the past few decades.

A final group of for-profit organizations that are often forgotten, although they are clearly forces for development and change in the health care field and offer a wealth of managerial challenges, are the commercial firms. Examples are pharmacies, drug manufacturers, clinical laboratories, investment bankers, and insurance companies. It is tempting to include in this group virtually any organization that employs a large number of people and thus is obligated to expend significant resources on health benefits. For example, at a health care conference several years ago in Detroit, a senior official of General Motors astounded the audience when he stated that his organization incurred a bill for health benefits in excess of $660 million dollars. Clearly such a stake in health care must produce an interest in streamlining the system.

THE NOT-FOR-PROFIT SECTOR

The not-for-profit organizations are those most often associated with the health field. Not for profit does not literally mean that the organization should not make a profit but rather that any surplus of revenue over expenses should not inure or be passed on to any group of stockholders or owners. Rather, all "profit" should be reinvested in the organization for its growth and development. Technically, such organizations are classified by the Internal Revenue Service as 501C3, which means not-for-profit and tax-exempt. They can be the recipients of tax-deductible contributions and do not pay sales or real estate taxes. Most community hospitals, health system agencies, hospital councils, and voluntary health-related organizations, such as the American Cancer Society or the Association for Voluntary Sterilization, are in the not-for-profit category, as are the Blue Cross and Blue Shield Plans throughout the United States.

Somewhat confusing within this framework is the mixed for-profit/not-for-profit situation of some organizations. Kaiser presents one of the simplest examples. The not-for-profit Kaiser hospitals work hand in glove with for-profit Permanente medical groups. A different type of example can be observed within a community hospital where a snack bar or gift shop is run on a for-profit basis and the surplus from this unit is used to subsidize the operations of other parts of the institution.

GOVERNMENT

The third large grouping of organizations is sponsored by the government. Official health agencies such as health departments or the U.S. Department of Health and Human Services (HHS) are the first to come to mind. Also in this category are the chain of Veterans Administration Hospitals and outpatient clinics (more recently renamed medical centers); military and public health service programs such as the Indian Health Service, municipally-owned hospitals and clinics, and state psychiatric facilities; and smaller organizations such as State

Health Care Coordinating Councils. Finally, there is a range of state health-related programs that often do not belong to official "health" agencies, such as family planning services, Medicaid management, and health care in prisons and jails.

MANAGERIAL MATRIX

The managerial matrix is a way of considering the issues in this chapter. Across the horizontal axis of the matrix are the three previously discussed classifications: for profit, not for profit, and government. The vertical axis lists a range of managerial functions and structural elements that relate to a manager's ability to organize and direct an organization.

Organizational Function

Delivery of Services

The first question considered in this matrix is that of primary function. What is it that the organization is supposed to do? One function is the delivery of services to individuals, and this clearly can and does occur in all three organizational forms. Abortion services are perhaps a simple illustration. An individual desiring such a service can usually find it in a not-for-profit hospital, for-profit abortion clinic, and in some states government-owned hospitals. Whether potential customers recognize the particular financial status of the organization they are dealing with is a matter of conjecture, as are some of the implications of the form. In some cases, however, it is an important distinction. For example, in Massachusetts, there is a state-licensed free-standing surgical center, a facility that provides one-day surgery and takes patients who are covered by a commercial insurance company or are willing to pay out of pocket for the operation. Blue Cross has been unwilling to cover its subscribers for this service; thus, the consumer with Blue Cross who is unwilling to foot the bill personally must go to a local hospital for the procedure at a price significantly higher than that at the surgical center. As a for-profit organization responsible to stockholders, the surgical center simply has no alternative but to refuse to accept the patient who is unwilling (or whose insurer is unwilling) to pay the bill. If it were a government or not-for-profit surgical center, it might view its responsibilities to the uncovered patient somewhat more generously.

Planning

A second possible organizational function is planning services. Does an organization have as its major responsibility the planning of health services? Most planning in the United States is carried out by governmental and nonprofit organizations. Indeed, the notion of profit suggests a special interest that is somewhat antithetical to the perceived value-free orientation of planning. Government is also in the business of planning, and many health care planning organizations function directly or indirectly as an arm of government. It should be noted that government, because of its power of licensure and control over vast sums of money, has the greatest potential leverage in planning health services. Private firms do enter the world of planning but usually as consultants to voluntary and government agencies that have the responsibility and authority for planning.

Monitoring and Evaluation

A third broad function is related to the monitoring and evaluation of health services. Clearly, this is a function that all organizations perform, but the question is really whether this is a primary function of the organization. Few proprietary organizations are empowered with the responsibility for monitoring or evaluating; in fact, this function is usually considered governmental in nature and sometimes is taken on in quasi-governmental organizations or voluntary organizations that receive most (if not all) of their funding from the government and thus are in one way or another accountable to government. Health Systems Agencies (HSAs) and Professional Standards Review Organizations (PSROs) are two cases in point. Both organizations were primarily developed as nongovernmental organizations; as prime contractors with the government, however, they in fact do follow government rules and regulations. A simple illustration of this is the HSA salary scale, which must be in compliance with HHS regulations.

There are some instances when proprietary organizations, particularly consulting firms, do get into the business of monitoring and evaluating health services. Recently, many of the large public accounting firms and management consulting firms have developed significant capabilities in the areas of health services. No longer do these firms limit themselves to the roles of auditor and occasional advisor. Today, these firms bid on requests for proposals from Washington or any state capital. Indeed, many of these firms have developed a remarkably strong record of excellent evaluations of health services.

Regulation

A fourth broad function is that of regulation. Government at the local, state, or national level has maintained the essential control; it could even be argued that this control can never be totally delegated or transferred. To a limited extent, however, governmental agencies transfer or allow voluntary agencies to "regulate." In Medicaid, for example, one level of government may subcontract with another level. In New York State, the health department of New York City was given a subcontract to pay and regulate Medicaid. A subsequent change in state government resulted in a different local agency being responsible—but never did the state totally abandon its control. At a national level, the federal government has transferred one of its major control devices for Medicare to the Joint Commission on Accreditation of Hospitals (JCAH) by allowing hospitals approved by this voluntary organization to participate in Medicare without further federal inspections. This pattern of cooperation among various levels of government and voluntary agencies appears to function as an organizational analogue of professional self-policing, and for the most part abuses have been limited.

The proprietary and voluntary self-interest groups have been excluded from these regulatory activities. However, it would be erroneous to conclude that they play no role—as consultants and political forces they play a vital role.

Proprietary, voluntary, and governmental organizations all pay for services, but each approaches payment with a rather different philosophy. The largest group of proprietary payers are the commercial insurance companies whose primary responsibility is to their stockholders. This "bottom line" approach, which takes into account the fact that insurance coverage is not marketed solely as a social good but also as a means for a commercial organization to make a profit, results in a somewhat hands-off attitude toward the health system and its consumers. The insurance company is duty bound to charge premiums in accordance with likely risks; if the costs of doing business go up, so do the premiums. To most outsiders, it appears that the big payer for health services is the voluntary Blue Cross organization. Blue Cross is actually a federation of scores of smaller Blue Cross plans located throughout the United States, each with an affiliation to the Chicago-based Blue Cross Association. These not-for-profit organizations have in recent years taken on an activist role in the health system in an effort to control costs and function as consumer advocates, particularly in regard to quality of services. Blue Cross and Blue Shield have been involved in research on the delivery of health services and the development of such programs as second opinion for surgery and health maintenance organizations (some private insurance carriers have also developed such programs).

Clearly, though, the largest bulk purchaser and the organization with the greatest financial leverage is the federal government, which, through its Medicare insurance plan and Medicaid program, has the ability to reshape the health system.

Goal Clarity

Another basic question is, How clear or diffuse are goals for organizations under these three classifications? In the for-profit organization, regardless of its function, the goal is clearly to make a profit. While it is evident that many for-profit organizations have "lines" that do not make a profit but may serve a public good, the organization's viability overall is quite clearly related to its ability to generate profits. A proprietary hospital or group practice cannot continue in existence if its charges are less than its costs; further, it will have significant difficulties if it cannot offer a balance sheet or profit-and-loss statement attractive enough to attract additional capital.

The not-for-profit organization has goals that are somewhat less clear. When asked what the goals of the hospital are, a typical teaching hospital administrator is likely to respond, "We have a threefold mission—teaching, research, and service." Not very often do these administrators talk of fiscal integrity, return on investments, or market penetration.

At another point on the spectrum of clear to diffuse goals are those of government health care organizations. In part, these organizations are constrained (or facilitated) because they are governmental agencies and must to a great extent be responsive to an elusive constituency; secondly, as public health organizations, they are constrained by the myriad problems that health care organizations of all types encounter.

In operational terms, these differences can be seen in the staffing ratios of proprietary hospitals versus those of government institutions. For example, in New York City in the mid-1970s, municipal hospitals had a ratio of seven staff to each bed (7.5:1), which was more than 100 percent higher than that of comparable proprietary or voluntary institutions. Analyses of the functioning of these institutions did not reveal any significant differences in patient mix or intensity of service; they did reveal lower productivity in the public sector, less control of productivity, more politically motivated appointments, and, finally, the anathema of all government programs—civil service, or what some view as the protection of incompetents or unnecessary staff. Return on investment decisions were not made on any basis other than political expediency. Another way of viewing this was offered by a former director of a government hospital when he referred to his institution as an employer of last resort in the community.

Revenues

How do these organizations earn or acquire their operating and capital funds? Proprietary organizations have only one significant source of operating capital, and that is from those who utilize their services. Fundamentally, these organizations become directly responsible to consumers, who in classical market terms vote with their dollars. Here it is necessary to recognize the clear imperfections of the medical care marketplace in that effective demand is for the most part determined by the providers, since consumers have quite limited knowledge of the costs and benefits of the various options. A group practice that is poorly located or offers services at inconvenient times may find itself out of business, however, simply because it depends on clients for revenue and has no opportunity to generate revenue from nonclient sources.

Capital funds are a somewhat different matter, since proprietary organizations can readily avail themselves of a range of private investors who willingly offer capital if they envision a good return on their investment. Perhaps the best example of this is the "hot" health care stocks of the mid-1970s. Indeed, major drug companies and health care equipment manufacturers still rank as blue chip or almost blue chip investments.

Not-for-profit organizations derive their operating funds from two major sources: consumers and philanthropy. In a very real sense, they too must satisfy their constituency; otherwise, their major source of operating income could be jeopardized. They have important ways of supplementing their accounts, however, such as fund-raising and gifts of various sorts. Such donations are rarely made to a proprietary organization, partly because these organizations do not solicit donations and partly because such a gift not only has no tax benefits for the donor but also is considered taxable income for the recipient. Further, few charitable organizations will provide money to for-profit organizations, since such gifts could jeopardize their own charitable status.

A third source of income is really not income at all but is essentially a bonus to not-for-profit organizations, and this is the tax exemption. Depending on location and quality of facility, a small community hospital may be worth millions of dollars. What would that amount to in terms of real estate tax? What about sales tax? If a medium-sized hospital with a $10 million budget, $6.5 million of which is for salaries and the rest is in supplies and material, has to pay a five percent tax on that $3.5 million, it is suddenly strapped with an additional expense of $175,000.

Government organizations and, to some extent, the quasi-governmental organizations acquire their money from three primary sources: consumers, philanthropy, and taxes. An HSA, for example, does not have to generate any funds itself (although some enrich their operations by seeking additional nongovernmental funding); its dollars flow from the federal budget, which is in turn related to taxes. Many government-funded programs, including those that are direct service programs, are removed from direct responsibility for generating their budgets. The conceptual notion of a service responsibility predominates, although even in government programs accountability is required; but this accountability is usually upward to a field or regional office as opposed to downward to the consumer.

A related question with regard to resources is, To what extent can managers affect the flow of resources into an organization? How much freedom does a manager have in developing programs to attract new clients or new dollars? Despite the range of controls exercised on health organizations, there is some degree of freedom; it varies in the three major types of organizations, however.

Managers in the for-profit operations probably have the greatest flexibility within their organizations for expanding revenue sources, since the clear mission of these organizations is related to their ability to generate adequate (and increased) revenues. Not-for-profit organizations have certain constraints, the most significant of which (as was noted earlier) is their tax-exempt status. While this is fundamentally a benefit, it is also a potential problem in that it may preclude the development of new and profitable services. This is not to suggest that not-for-profit organizations cannot or do not go out and market their services—indeed they do in a variety of ways. Perhaps the major conceptual constraint is related to the somewhat more diffuse mission of the not-for-profit organization; thus, a not-for-profit organization might knowingly develop a program that is clearly unlikely to be self-supporting simply because there is a community need for it or because it is viewed as part of the organization's service responsibility. Rarely is such benevolent behavior seen in for-profit organizations.

Government organizations are usually much more constrained than either of the two other types of organizations. Government organizations may be prevented by law or custom from offering services to "noneligible" recipients—or, to put it another way, the programs in which they are engaged are developed solely to satisfy certain clearly defined constituencies. To go beyond those constituencies is an encroachment on someone else's territory and may be beyond their scope of responsibilities and likely reimbursement. If an organization does go beyond its jurisdiction, there are often disincentives to provide the service. For example, many governmental hospitals that provided care to Blue Cross subscribers in the past could not be reimbursed by Blue Cross for the service, nor (theoretically) could they be reimbursed from their home agencies; yet they had to utilize their resources to provide that care.

Expenses

While resources are one managerial headache, costs are no doubt the major headache of managers of all health care organizations. The question of concern here is, To what extent can managers in these various organizations control costs? To address this question properly, it must be recognized that the typical health care organization has two types of costs: fixed and variable. The fixed costs are those which, for the most part, are beyond the scope of the organization's, or at least the manager's, ability to control and may be considered overhead. Of course, even this concept is a bit illusory, since there is a certain latitude within fixed costs; for example, energy costs might be considered fixed, and yet through careful analysis of alternative systems a manager might find satisfactory substitutes. The variable costs are simply those attached to each specific visit. As an illustration, a family planning clinic has fixed costs for its land and building (mortgages and interest), regardless of the number of visits of patients per week, month, or year; however, each visit generates other costs directly related to the visits, such as supplies that are consumed.

The single largest item in virtually any health care budget is salaries, typically running upwards of 60 percent in a hospital. How can a manager affect that item? In a for-profit enterprise, the traditional solution is careful attention to productivity and hiring. Control of this critical section of the budget has been more difficult, however, in government and voluntary agencies where hiring has been used to provide a safety valve for unemployment. In one of the more blatant exercises of this practice, the Veterans Administration curtailed hiring in 1978, which had the net effect of freezing institutions at the present employment levels and forcing them to hire more part-time workers rather than full-time workers. The "public relations effect" was a decrease in unemployment, but the individual worker had less security and certainly less money.

Community organizations, simply because of their "closeness" with the community, must be more circumspect in how they deal with this issue of staffing. Perhaps one of the best examples is the Hunterdon Medical Center, where in the mid-1970s, in response to a declining census, they closed off beds—which logically would have dictated the laying off of workers. Yet, as one of its largest employers, the hospital felt a responsibility to the community and decided not to lay off workers, hence putting itself into a difficult financial situation. Would a for-profit company have acted in such a way?

Recently, one of the nation's largest tire manufacturers negotiated a 50 cents per hour pay decrease with its union so that the plant would not follow other companies that have moved to the Sun Belt and abandoned workers to the "decaying" industrial East. Could this happen in the health care field? How will New York City close down 5,000 hospital beds without losing 15,000 jobs? Most managers admit that their health care organizations are overstaffed, but what can they do about it? In the for-profit organization, the answers seem simpler, perhaps because the self-interest of the organization is more clearly identified than the amorphous "public interest" that the government or voluntary organization must serve.

Feedback and Action

Assuming that the problem has been diagnosed, then what can be done? This is perhaps one of the most perplexing problems facing the on-line manager. In the context of the matrix, this is termed the feedback loop and action. To what extent will data and analysis result in some type of corrective action? Using a personnel example again, assume that a particular program area is not achieving its goals because an individual worker is simply and blatantly unproductive. Attempts at assisting the worker have been to no avail, and the manager has come to the distasteful conclusion that the worker must be fired. In the for-profit organization, it is usually the manager's prerogative to discharge the worker; if justification is required, it is to a higher level manager or perhaps a union. In the voluntary agency, additional constraints may be imposed because of community pressure— discharging an informal community leader may bring unacceptable consequences. In government, the obvious problem is the civil service, a system that was designed to protect the worker from arbitrary and capricious "bosses" and that now functions, in part, to protect arbitrary and capricious workers from the reasonable and often difficult economic decisions of management.

Many other examples can be used to illustrate the differences among these three major organization types when they are faced with data and information. In New York City, the president of the Health and Hospitals Corporation "buried" a report on one of his hospitals because he felt the community would be outraged if it was known that "their" hospital was threatened with closing. A for-profit management company "cleaned house" at Roosevelt Hospital in New York by laying off hundreds of employees and thus brought a measure of fiscal stability to that institution. Is it possible that the former hospital director, one of the nation's most thoughtful and knowledgeable professionals, had simply not been aware of the solution? Hardly! Rather, as the agent of a charitable organization, he was really not empowered to make the "hard-nosed" business decisions that were acceptable under the regime of a proprietary business firm.

Action then is in large part related to the number of constituencies that must be satisfied. Certain organizations have fewer constituencies than others, and the goals of some are sharper than others. Action for the for-profit organization relates to the bottom line—today or in the foreseeable future; at the other extreme, action in government relates to an unclear and oft debated public good, as well as to the prospect of reappointment or reelection.

MANAGERIAL TIME FRAME

The time frame in which management must act may differ in these various organizational arrangements. In for-profit and voluntary organizations, it is postulated that both top and middle management have and can afford a time frame long enough to plan and implement properly. In essence, they can emulate the model of private industry, such as the automobile industry in which up to a decade may pass from the time of a new model's inception to the time of its introduction. Indeed, even in these times of "future shock," Iacocca, the new president of Chrysler, admitted in late 1978 that his real impact on the company would not be felt until 1982.

Both top and middle management have a sense of stability that allows them to plan, develop, and, in some cases, test alternatives. They simply do not have to have a "splash" to survive the next political purge or election.

For the middle manager in government, who is often protected by civil service, the time frame may also be long. On the other hand, top management in governmental agencies and programs are continually asked to produce results by absurd deadlines. A governor is elected in November and asked to produce a multi-billion dollar budget in January. A congressman complains, and a secretary or commissioner is asked to solve a complicated social problem within a few days.

Both facilitating and complicating these public management positions is the press. Most people cannot name the heads of the Fortune 500 companies but can easily identify senior government officials. Why? Because these officials are always in the spotlight and, in many senses, are being asked for "action." A government agency must act in order to develop a constituency both within and outside of government and thus ensure its own managerial well-being. Private and voluntary organizations simply do not have to be concerned with the nourishing of such constituencies for their resources and can afford more independence, both in planning and action.

The reward structure for management is rather diffuse and sometimes confusing. In the private and not-for-profit organizations, income, benefits, and privileges are usually directly related to the quality and quantity of work—or, to put it another way, to the value or esteem in which the organization holds a person. A top manager in one of these two organization types has considerable latitude in how or when people are rewarded; sometimes a day off, a small bonus, or a new title can be given. For top management in the government organizations, however, degrees of freedom are severely limited, particularly with nonprofessional staff. With so little latitude, managers may find themselves not only unable to motivate employees but also unable to prevent them from being dissatisfied because of those tremendous trivialities that so often irritate employees and prevent them from doing a reasonable day's work.

THE MANAGEMENT ROLE

In both the private and voluntary organizations, individuals become managers and remain managers because of their loyalty and performance. Most organizations want people who are loyal to their ideas, concepts, and goals. Loyalty is not enough, however. The manager must have needed skills, which can range from those of being a financially technocratic whiz to being a skilled negotiator. Organizations have natural histories and needs for different types of people at different times. The manager's skills must contribute to the organization, and the possessor must be recognized as the integral implementer of the skills.

In a theoretical sense, it could be argued that effective health administrators are those who have an understanding of the health system within which they have to operate, the skills to manage it, and the knowledge to apply those skills judiciously. Some, on the other hand, argue that "management is management" and is a totally transferable skill. Others say that "management is a bunch of crap" and that what a manager really needs is to know something about how health services are organized and to have a feel for the "people."

The most costly and possibly most unfortunate natural experiment on this issue has been the New York City Health and Hospitals Corporation. In 1978, the newly appointed president of this billion dollar corporation was described by the mayor as a man with top-flight management skills gleaned from his experiences as the number two man in the New York City Police Department. The official health establishment in New York City mumbled under its breath and did nothing. Who did this management expert replace?—a former Catholic priest and college chaplain who, by a series of accidents, became president of the corporation with less than five years in health administration (not one day of which amounted to anything approximating hospital administration). Who had he replaced?—an outspoken activist physician without a day's worth of hospital administration experience who had replaced a psychiatrist with federal government experience but no hospital administration experience.

In this natural experiment, it has been demonstrated that the road to the top in government has nothing to do with a logical model of managerial competency and experience but rather political expediency. Those appointed for such reasons are obligated to those with the appointment power. Thus, in order to stay on the top in a political position, those appointed must pay extremely careful attention to constituencies, not only their own, but, perhaps more importantly, those of the individuals who have the power to appoint (and no doubt) remove them.

CONCLUSION

Each of the three types of organizations appeals to different constituencies, has different possibilities to offer to a public, and, in this author's opinion, has an appropriate role in the health system. Ideologues would claim that the poor can be served properly only in the public general hospital because that is the institution where there is an accountability. How has this accountability been brought into play? Certainly not in the accessibility, availability, or even quality of services. If there is accountability in these institutions, it appears to be related more to the workers than to the patients. Private health care organizations are criticized for "skimming the cream" of the system; however, they have also reacted much more rapidly and in some respects more sensitively to public needs. When the abortion laws were passed, where were the public clinics and voluntary agencies, for example? The "Medicaid mill" is criticized—but who else is willing to go into Washington Heights or the South Bronx and provide care? Finally, voluntary organizations are criticized for virtually everything, but it must be remembered that they have made major contributions to progress in clinical medicine and to the advancement of health care.

In sum, the United States has a pluralistic system that has many edges and angles that disturb and perturb—but, before we throw it out, it behooves us to understand it and make it work in the most effective way for the special needs of our society.

CASE STUDY

Developing an HMO*

In the late 1950s, State University faced an escalating problem with its health services for students. Utilization was less than half the mean for residential colleges, reflecting widespread student dissatisfaction, and many students either sought care from local private practitioners or went home ill. The staff attitude had been reported as "You're going to be sick for a week or so; why don't you go home?" At the same time, State University enrollment was expected to increase rapidly in the 1960s as the effects of the postwar baby boom reached the college population. In 1958, the university received a capital appropriation for a new infirmary, and in 1959 it convened a Board of Visitors, composed of local practitioners, alumni, university administrators, and college health professionals from other institutions, to design a health program appropriate to the needs of the growing student body and the anticipated new facility. The staff of the health service were not included on the Board of Visitors but were offered an opportunity to present their ideas and opinions before the board. The following year, Dr. John Smith was appointed director of health services. Smith, a family practitioner in town who saw many students from the university, had acquired a clear picture of a new direction for the health services as a member of the Board of Visitors.

Smith faced some serious problems in his new position. The previous senior physician's retirement blunted some of the anxiety of the remaining staff, but they still saw the new director as a serious threat to their security because of his reputed attitude of "softness" to students (he had been the refuge of many who had been dissatisfied with campus medical services). Students, in general, had developed a strong distrust for the university's concern for their health. The remaining staff held an equally strong distrust for students and their motives for seeking health care. Finally, the state personnel system seriously limited the possibility of replacing staff members because of both job security regulations and salary levels for physicians and other professionals that were significantly below those of other similar positions.

Progress, which was slow at first but accelerated with time, was made possible because of two significant conditions. First, in 1961, a student health fee was established, designed to be the revenue source for professional staff salaries. Holding these fees in a special account, rather than depositing them in the state treasury, made it possible to escape the state salary limit for physicians. It also established the important principle of direct accountability of the health program to students (as well as to the administration) and gave Smith the opportunity to

---

*This case study was prepared by Robert Gage, M.D., Professor of Public Health, University of Massachusetts at Amherst.

develop a constituency that could affirm or deny support for the expanding program. Second, the university began a period of unprecedented growth, increasing its enrollment by 1,500 students per year during the ten-year period beginning in 1962. This both broadened the financial base for support and readily justified an even more rapid recruitment of staff, who came on board committed to providing high quality preventive medicine and services oriented to the student population.

As the quality of care and the attitude of the staff toward students improved, there were opportunities, even requests, to broaden the range of services. An active mental health program was begun in 1961, an environmental health and safety program in 1964, and health education in 1967. A student request for dental service had to be deferred until an addition to the new infirmary could be opened in 1974. Students were involved actively in program planning and service assessment, and the program was viewed as successful by all parameters of measurement.

The one area in which Smith failed was in a 1963 proposal to bring student dependents into the program. He attended a special meeting of the district medical society, where he found that the previous level of trust he had enjoyed with professional colleagues had broken down. He was advised that the university's only appropriate role in dependent care was to support an insurance or other plan that would ensure payment to local practitioners for services rendered to dependents. This was occurring at a time when there was intense national pressure, generated by the American Medical Association, opposing any governmental intrusion into the delivery of medical services. The university's medical staff was too small a minority in the medical society to gain support for a program that threatened local physicians, and no compromise position had been prepared.

During the late 1960s, it became apparent to faculty members that students were receiving health care with which they seemed satisfied (in contrast to most schools, where the health service shares with the dining service the dubious distinction of being the chief object of student criticism) and at a cost substantially below comparable service from the private sector. Those who had received on-campus emergency care bore testimony to its effectiveness and convenience. This opportunity became increasingly attractive as the cost of care rose and as out-of-hours and emergency care became more difficult to obtain in the vicinity.

In 1970, the University Faculty Senate voted "to go on record as supporting a study of possible extension and reorganization of the health program for the University community." The vote directed attention to a prepaid group practice as a means of providing "a wide range of health services." A faculty-student-staff-administration committee was formed to study the problem. Among members of the committee were the assistant director of the health services, a member of the public health faculty, a member of the industrial engineering faculty, and a member of the school of business faculty whose special interest was health insurance. All were staunch supporters of a prepaid group practice.

During the spring of 1971, the committee reported its solid endorsement of the prepaid group practice, noting that it "is desirable and appears feasible." The senate accepted the report and recommended a continuation of the feasibility study. This action, based on more complete information than the first, constituted a solid endorsement by the faculty governance body and served notice that the recommendation was not to be taken lightly. It came at a time when faculty prerogatives were being asserted more stridently and the Faculty Senate was becoming increasingly determined not to permit its recommendations to be over-looked by the administration.

The action did, however, raise some serious questions about a facility currently supported almost entirely by students, in which students, faculty, staff, and their dependents would receive services concurrently:

1. How could student-faculty competition for services be avoided? How could students be assured that faculty and/or staff would not receive preferential treatment?
2. How could a larger clientele be served in a facility that already was seriously overcrowded by students? A major addition had been promised but had not progressed beyond preliminary planning.
3. Could financing be separated with sufficient clarity to assure students that they were not financing faculty care, or vice versa?
4. How could the relatively heavy cost of a student dependents' program be financed?

The committee resumed its planning with renewed energy in the light of this endorsement and the knowledge that the addition to the campus health center had received final approval from the state building authority. One of its moves was to contact the White Medical Group, a small private fee-for-service group practice, to determine what, if any, interest it had in joint planning. Its director indicated a lack of interest in new service delivery projects, and he declined the committee's invitation to join the new project.

In January, 1972, the committee made its final report, which contained a detailed enumeration of benefits from a prepaid group practice for the university community, drew attention to similar plans in operation at Harvard and Yale, and made estimates of cost, which were favorable in comparison with the concurrent health insurance plan for state employees. It recommended "strongly" that steps be taken to implement the plan in the near future. The Faculty Senate accepted the report and for the third time went on record as favoring action. The last two votes had been without audible dissent.

THE WHITE MEDICAL GROUP

The White Medical Group was formed in the mid 1960s when Dr. Robert White took on a partner and moved to a newly constructed set of offices. The plan of the founders was to have a group practice in which family practitioners formed the nucleus, supported by part-time specialists and ancillary services. The concept was well accepted in the community, and services offered at the center grew steadily during the next three years to include pediatrics, dentistry, laboratory services, and part-time internal medicine.

Late in 1968, the group was joined by Dr. Alvin Green, and from then on it began to expand much more dramatically. Green had been a member of the medical staff of the university during 1964-1966 and had left to develop an emergency-outpatient service at a hospital in a neighboring community. His success there was notable; but the hospital's trustees ultimately became uncomfortable with his vision, and he left to join the White Medical Group where developmental opportunities seemed rich. The university, and with it the population of the university city area, was expanding with no end in sight. Green was dedicated to group practice and saw the university employees as a population likely to be congenial to his interests. Before he joined White, he and Smith had discussed the possibility of setting up a health center for employees, but he was disheartened by Smith's assessment of the minimum time it would take to marshall support and to get the plan in operation.

In 1969-1970, soon after he had assumed leadership of the White Medical Group and demonstrated its growth potential, Green initiated discussions with Blue Shield regarding its sponsorship of a prepaid group practice. The extent of proposed coverage originally discussed with Blue Shield remains uncertain. The White Medical Group budget submitted as part of the certificate-of-need request projected a first year income of $360,000 from the group practice's fee-for-service patients and $160,000 from 2,000 prepaid patients being charged $80 per year. The discussions were cordial, tentative, and intermittent. It was apparent to Green, however, that Blue Shield was unlikely to offer any commitment of solid support in either risk money or marketing guarantees, at least not within the time frame he was projecting for development. Separate preliminary discussions were equally unfruitful with Blue Cross, which apparently did most of the marketing for Blue Shield, yet remained in a separate organization. In evaluating these tepid responses, two factors should be kept in mind. First, Blue Cross was assessing its experiences with the prepaid plan in another university community in a different part of the state. In that experience, the Blue Cross agreement to provide marketing guarantees had been costly, but the extent of losses was uncertain. Second, it seemed apparent that Blue Shield at least, which was heavily dependent for its vigor upon the blessing of the state medical society, was adopting a cautious watch-and-wait stance toward prepaid plans that differed from the medical foundation approach supported by the medical society (and which preserved the fee-for-service principle).

The White Medical Group experienced phenomenal growth under Green's energetic and imaginative leadership and projected comparable growth for the future. In 1972, it reported a three-year increase in its "active" records from 5,000 to 16,000, yet its staff had increased to six full-time and three part-time physicians, plus dentists and laboratory services. It was looking toward the formation of a large multispecialty group that would be the major medical care provider for the area. Opportunities for additional growth were constrained by serious crowding in its present building, but there was room for expansion, so plans for building were begun. In March, 1972, the White Medical Group presented its plan for a major building program to the Regional Health Planning Council, the "b" agency that could recommend a certificate of need.

THE REGIONAL HEALTH PLANNING COUNCIL

In 1971, independent of the university or the White Medical Group, the Regional Health Planning Council made a survey of health resources in that part of the state and found that the area was short 19 physicians relative to nationally recommended standards. In addition, it noted that, since adjacent counties were also short and since several physicians identified in the survey confined their services to institutional practice, the actual shortage was probably greater than that reported.

In 1972, however, when White Medical Group made its request for a certificate of need, the council was uneasy about granting it, especially since it knew that the university was making active plans for a similar development. Before acting officially on the request, the council asked the university and the White Medical Group, who now were obviously in open competition, to come together with a joint plan upon which the certificate-of-need application could be judged more objectively. The result was a letter of intent; in June, 1972, both groups agreed for a period of one year to work for a mutually satisfactory solution. By imposing this condition, the council apparently hoped to give each an opportunity to grow appropriately without preempting the prerogatives of the other and, in so doing, to work out some sharing of expensive resources that otherwise would have to be duplicated, e.g., x-ray/fluorographic equipment. The council acted in spite of an emotional petition from many members of the district medical society against supporting the White Medical Group's application.

THE UNIVERSITY ADMINISTRATION

From the beginning, the university administration had been cool in its response to the faculty's interest in an expanded health program. Although the student health program had gained great respect, both on campus and nationally, the administration felt a persistent uneasiness with the success Smith had achieved in developing student support for the program; this was in spite of the fact that, except for the environmental health service, it was funded entirely by students.

In 1971, as part of a number of changes in the top administration on campus, William Jones, a member of the biology faculty, was appointed as the first vice chancellor for student affairs. Jones had had over 20 years of service as scientist and administrator at the National Institutes of Health before coming to the university and had developed uncanny political intuition in addition to bureaucratic caution. One year later, the chancellor resigned. Jones was appointed chancellor, and he asked Smith to become vice chancellor for student affairs. The health service was one of the responsibilities of student affairs.

Smith was succeeded as director of health services by Mr. Harvey Singer, who had been in charge of administration for the health service and was serving on the Faculty Senate study committee. Appointment of a nonphysician to head the health services created some potentially serious anxiety among some members of the medical staff, which now numbered 13 full-time physicians (in addition to a mental health professional staff of 8). It aroused latent staff suspicion that their interests would not be held paramount in responding to the faculty request for care. This internal dissension turned out to be one of the most disturbing (and least justified) difficulties with which Singer had to contend in developing plans for the health maintenance organization (HMO).

Despite Smith's easy access to Chancellor Jones, the staff of the president's office, and the trustees, it appeared that, as faculty interest in health services increased, Jones' serious reservations started surfacing.

1. Could faculty be attended without compromising services to students—or, equally important, without *appearing* to compromise student welfare?
2. Why should the university, which had a presumed primary mission related to education, become involved unnecessarily in a service program for a group that should be able to take care of itself?
3. What would be the eventual cost of this extension of service: capital, maintenance, service (e.g., parking)?

Both Smith and Singer were convinced that the first objective could be resolved. Singer had worked long and patiently with the Student Health Advisory Board and assured Smith that all potential areas of conflict had been resolved. A key feature of the assurance was the success of the computerized appointment system, which had demonstrated to students that appointments could be made objectively and that waiting time could be reduced without compromising the availability of urgent care. In substance, therefore, this objection could be dismissed. On the other hand, it was an emotion-laden issue to which every student responded each time it was raised.

The mission of the institution, on the other hand, was an ideological issue with as many potential resolutions as there were interest groups. In general, the administration had tried to finesse involvement in or commitment to nonessential activities, especially any that might polarize interest groups or lead to any assumption of responsibility for unnecessary or distracting activities. Fiscal austerity was threatened. The faculty was reacting to the development of a president's office in the state capital and a perception that power was being taken from the campus; faculty were also being courted by prospective collective bargaining agents. Smith had argued in the past that health service and educational activities could not be divorced; he now asserted that the university had social responsibilities in the area of service that it could ill-afford to overlook. He was strongly supported in this area by members of the president's staff, some of whom were deeply interested in the proposed HMO but reluctant to interfere prematurely in on-campus discussions.

There was no immediate answer to Jones' third question, beyond an assurance that no capital outlay would be required and any hidden maintenance costs would be balanced by improvement in faculty/staff morale and productivity. The assurance was less than fully convincing.

In light of the January, 1972, action of the Faculty Senate and the June, 1972, agreement, Jones was in the position of having to demonstrate the administration's support for continued planning or face increasing faculty hostility. One important component of this unfolding drama was that Jones and Green had been close neighbors, and Green was Jones' physician. On the basis of his own experience, Green was of the opinion that the university was incapable of making a timely and effective response to the faculty's request. In addition, another university physician who was opposed personally to the HMO had been Jones' next-door neighbor and obviously nourished the chancellor's anxieties.

JOINT PLANNING FOR THE HMO

Following execution of the letter of intent, Jones met with Smith, Singer, and some members of the study committee to reach an accord about the direction and extent of the next steps. Although his concerns had not all been resolved completely, he did agree to authorize a joint application for a grant for a more detailed feasibility study, but with the clear understanding that no final approval could be inferred. The result was an application to the Regional Medical Program for planning funds. A grant of $23,052 was awarded in March, 1973, and a private health care consulting firm was employed to carry out the project. In the meantime, the White Group had begun building, amid speculation about whether or not it would adhere to the agreement beyond the one year specified: it had its building and was under increasing pressure from local physicians to withdraw from the HMO.

The consultant's market survey of the area confirmed the impression of need for considerable additional health care and of substantial interest in the prepaid group practice. The study also reviewed in detail the unique legal problems confronting a public institution in working with a private provider. As the study proceeded, confidence increased in the feasibility of forming an HMO that would utilize both White and the university as alternative service delivery sites. It came as no surprise, therefore, when the final report in July, 1974, identified no legal, organizational, or financial problems that could not be resolved. Its specific recommendation was to work for the formation of a HMO that would, in turn, contract for all services with the two groups.

The time of decision was at hand. Singer and Smith had kept the president's staff apprised of progress and had received considerable encouragement from them. The White Medical Group had completed its building and already was under some financial stress for a more reliable income. Its sharpened "business" orientation had created uneasiness among some of its clientele. In March, 1974, the University Health Council, which had supplanted the study committee as review body for health policy, reported solid endorsement of the developing plans. Endorsement was received also from the Faculty Senate (again!), the undergraduate and graduate student organizations, the association of nonacademic professional employees, and two collective bargaining units. In May, 1974, Singer and Smith made an informal presentation to the board of trustees, primarily to provide information but also to get a feeling for the level of support or opposition. The State Commissioner of Health (a university trustee) was very helpful in allaying anxiety, as he urged support for the plan. The consultants gave support in two crucial directions: (1) the proposal was declared sound and not beyond implementation in light of the HMO act of December, 1973, and (2) the proposal could be implemented only by a White and university "partnership"—neither could succeed alone.

In August, 1974, four years of planning was climaxed by Jones' agreement, with the president's knowledge, to approve the submission by the university and White of a grant application for $122,000 from the Department of Health, Education and Welfare for planning and development of the University Area Health Plan, which for the first time would bring together a public and a private provider in the structure of an HMO.

Discussion Questions

1. What would have happened had the White Medical Group's application for a certificate of need been supported?
2. How might things be different *or* have to be done differently if Smith was not vice chancellor?
3. What would be the anticipated problems of moving the HMO into the implementation stage?
4. How does the orientation and structure of White and the university likely affect their relationship on this project?

Chapter 4

Setting Objectives in the Health Industry

As noted in Chapter 3, different types of health care organizations have different fundamental goals or objectives, and these differing objectives can very much affect the managerial activities of the organization. In order to put these objectives into the perspective of the health system, it is necessary to establish a definition of system. Several popular ones include

- "an organization of interrelated and interdependent parts that form a unity."[1]

- "a set of parts coordinated to accomplish a set of goals."[2]

- "an organized or complex whole: an assemblage or combination of things or parts forming a complex or unitary whole."[3]

An illustration of systems is offered by a stereo set-up, which is likely to include a tuner-receiver, turntable, tape recorder, and speakers. Do they make a system? Not yet! They are the components of a system; they become a system only when the wires connecting all the components are set into place and the set is plugged into a power source. Within the system, there are components that are considerably more important than others—for example, while the breakdown of one speaker will affect the quality of sound, the other speaker's functioning will prevent a total system collapse. On the other hand, if the power transformer in the receiver blows out, the rest of the system becomes mute. In the system of the human body, it can also be seen how the breakdown of one leading component, such as the heart or brain, can result in a total shutdown; however, the breakdown of other components, such as sight, can be compensated for to an extent by the remainder of the system. In short, then, systems are comprised of interrelated components that must function together in order to achieve a desired outcome.

A diagram of the U.S. health system that was developed by the American Public Health Association illustrates its components and functioning (Figure 4-1).[4]

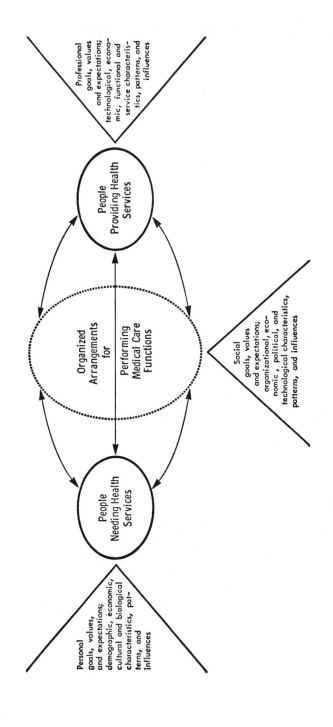

Figure 4-1 The Medical Care Complex: Boundaries

Source: American Public Health Association, *A Guide to Medical Care Administration, Vol. I, Concepts and Principles,* 1964, p. 15.

In brief, it notes that the system has three major components: (1) the personal component, i.e., individuals who need or demand health services; (2) the professional component, or the providers of services; and (3) the social component or the organizational arrangements for delivering the care. Each of these components is influenced by a host of factors, including individual values, beliefs, opinions, knowledge, and economics. For example, numerous authors have shown a differential use of health services based on ethnic backgrounds of patients; physicians in teaching hospitals tend to behave differently (for example, order more ancillary tests) than those in nonteaching hospitals; and finally, as Shain and Roemer noted over two decades ago, the availability of facilities and programs generates its own "business." [5,6,7]

REAL AND STATED GOALS

The fundamental question that must be dealt with is, What is the objective of the health system and its organizational components, such as hospitals, ambulatory care centers, and even physicians' offices? Is this objective to raise the health status of an individual or a community, or simply to deal with symptomatic problems? An answer to that question must begin with the realization that goals can be two things: real and stated. For example, most administrators of large health care facilities or programs say that they have three goals: teaching, research, and service. But what are the real goals? What do they actually mean when they say teaching, research, or service? What is behind such a goal?

The somewhat murky history of obstetrics in the United States might be used to illustrate this point. What was behind the stated goals of the physician leaders of this profession during the controversy that raged in the United States and Great Britain over the use of midwives in the late 1800s and early 1900s? The solution in Great Britain was the education, licensing, and upgrading of midwives to a position in the medical hierarchy whereby they would be able to deliver most normal babies. In the United States the controversy raged for years, pitting those physicians in the new specialty of obstetrics against midwives (a rather disorganized group). Even the American Medical Association had a surprising position on this issue. In 1912, its president, the noted physician Dr. Abraham Jacobi, pointed out in his inaugural address that the current view of nurse-midwives as dirty and sloppy women was based not on fact but rather conjecture and that, if the clinical facts surrounding obstetrical care were examined, physicians—not midwives—would be eliminated.[8]

What then motivated distinguished professors to work so assiduously to eliminate midwives? Was it simply that the midwife was providing medical care of a poorer quality? According to some sources, the goal was to eliminate midwives in order to provide the appropriate volume of patients for fledgling physicians to practice their new skills. Further, once these skills were learned, midwives had to be eliminated if physicians were to build a practice to support themselves. Others have argued that midwifery died because the new immigrants found seeing a physician the modern way, while midwifery was considered "old-fashioned."[9]

Regardless of the reason, it is obvious that midwifery essentially passed from the scene, even though there was no clearly defined medical care objective in its elimination. More recently, other public policy decisions in health care have been made with almost the same lack of clear objectives. A case in point might be house calls. As a matter of public and private policy, the house call has been eliminated. Was this a deliberate objective of the health system? Indeed, was it in the best interests of the health status of the individual and community, or rather in the best interests of the providers and/or the organized arrangements for delivering the services?[10]

The concept of prisons can also be used to illustrate the problem faced in determining real and stated goals. Many wardens, sheriffs, or court officers state that prison is a place for rehabilitation; others say that it is a place where offenders go to "pay their debt to society" or, to put it another way, it is a place for punishment. Essential to all of these stated goals is the real goal; a prison is an institution organized by society to segregate people from "free" society for some period of time. Although never overtly stated, one of the clearest goals of any prison or jail is that of keeping certain people locked up.

GOAL SETTING

It is useful to remember that goals are set in a variety of ways, and organizations often have multiple and sometimes conflicting goals; indeed, the manager is frequently charged with resolving the most serious of these conflicts.

In general, goals are set as a result of four major factors: (1) politics, (2) economics, (3) constituencies, and (4) organizational personalities. Politics are local, national, regional and environmental—that is, internal. For example, the sheriff and the mayor of a southern city realized that the health and medical conditions of a prison—which had already resulted in a federal lawsuit—would prove an embarrassing political issue during a forthcoming election unless the situation was "cleaned up." Further, they envisioned the possibility of amassing some political capital out of developing a model health system. Internally—that is, within the prison—the feeling was that the system was simply out of control and the warden and sheriff were being used for the political purposes of the medical department. Thus, to some extent, a desire for change was dictated as a convergence of local political needs. Legal factors accelerated these changes, but the essential elements for the goals were found in politics.[11]

Always an important factor, economics is becoming an even stronger element in the setting of organizational goals. In a small northeastern town, two competing hospitals are now attempting to resolve their differences so that a merger can be consummated. Why is there even an interest in this merger between hospitals that have traditionally been competitors and have somewhat different social orientations? The answer appears to be related to the difficulty of surviving economically in an increasingly regulated environment. Although neither institution is weak enough to be "picked off," neither has enough clout in the state capital to obtain a certificate of need or a rate increase. Together, they would move up a few notches in the hierarchy of institutions and could afford to take advantage of certain strategies that individually they can not afford, such as the use of expensive (and thought to be) effective consultants and more sophisticated financial planning. Finally, they believe that their combined organizations will allow for better sharing of services and a generally more efficient operation.

The conventional wisdom in health care is that the demand for services comes from inside, not from outside. The patient walks in, states a complaint and symptoms, and goes through the usual examination. Despite what the consumer may think or feel, the health professional "turns on" the effective demand of the system. The physician orders the laboratory tests, x-rays, back brace, or whatever. The only demand actually generated by the patient is through drugstores, herbalists, and such. To a large extent, this theory has been correct. In the past few years, however, there has been a slight change, and perhaps newer changes are in the offing. Organized patient constituencies are demanding services. A recent, clear example is abortion services. With the legalization of first trimester abortions, the patient walks into the medical facility and demands a specific service; she does not discuss a symptom and say "help me," but rather states in unequivocal language what medical procedure she wishes to obtain. Community groups have grown more vocal about their desires, and sometimes these desires, which are wrapped in the mantle of medical care, are only masking something else. For example, were the goals of neighborhood health centers to provide medical care or jobs?

Finally, it is imperative to recognize the importance of the individual in setting organizational goals. At the national level, a president can restate and reorganize national priorities. One person in a leadership position can have power and choose to exercise it. At a Veterans Administration Medical Center, for example, a new director may shift the goal of that seemingly highly controlled organization from that of being a self-sufficient non-community-oriented organization into that of being an organization that is an integral part of the economic and professional life of a community. Examples abound in the management literature about the role individuals can and do play in the leadership and management of organizations. These people not only set new and often exciting goals, but also they implement them and leave a permanent mark on the organization for having done so. The history of the Ford Motor Company demonstrates the power of organizational personalities in setting and effecting goals; the senior Mr. Ford built and then almost destroyed the company, and the younger Mr. Ford "saved" it.

While personalities can in fact change organizational goals, many organizations are like giant ocean liners and need time to make the shift; otherwise, they can run into extreme trouble. Again, as the Chrysler president commented, it will be four years before the impact of his changes can be clearly seen.

IDENTIFICATION OF ORGANIZATIONAL GOALS

Skeptics like to point out that the goals of most organizations predate the manager, often by that manager's lifetime; so why bother identifying organizational goals? There is really only one reason; it gives the new manager the necessary bearings to chart a suitable personal course in the organization. The identification of goals has value to the organization in three major ways: orientation, legitimization, and measurement.

Orientation

Goal identification provides an organization with a certain direction, or orientation, that can and does help in the shaping of planning and policy directions. In practice, however, most organizations, particularly health care ones it sometimes seems, have such general goals that they can and do fit into their plans whatever makes sense at a given time. To be less charitable, it could be said that most of these organizations are simply responding as typical economic opportunists. One health services research center began its career with a clear goal and orientation toward community health needs; even its name indicated a commitment to the community. In the early years of the research center, a great deal of effort and many dollars were funneled into identifying community needs and developing research projects that would meet these needs. Its goals during these early years were clearly very community oriented; because of initially secure funding from foundations that shared its goals, the center was able to pursue its community direction. As the initial grant funds were exhausted, however, the research center began searching for funds simply to pay staff and rent. Over time the orientation shifted from the community needs for which there were no funds to a variety of national problems for which funds were available. More recently, in response to the fact that private foundation funds are again available, the nature of the problems to be researched in this center has again shifted.

In practice, then, a major orientation of most organizations is simply survival; organizations do not commit suicide. When the March of Dimes met its goal of contributing to the conquest of polio, it did not close down its operation. Rather, it shifted its focus to a new "goal": birth defects.

Orientation should not be belittled; it has an important influence on the resources that are attracted to an organization. Managers who seek positions are or should be interested in the goals of the organization with which they are likely to be associated. Is there a shared orientation or general value system—how important is that issue? It might be of major consequence for the viability of an organization. For example, an excellent small rural hospital interested basically in maintaining its special niche as an excellent small rural hospital hired a director who misunderstood the goals of the hospital, or perhaps the hospital misunderstood its own goals when he was hired. With an evangelical burst of energy, the new director began to transform the institution into a national model of rural medicine. After less than a year, he was forced to resign—his goals and the institution's became irreconcilable. Had he known that the hospital was not interested in the "big time," he would not have considered the position—and maybe the hospital did not understand what the "big time" meant before the new director's regime.

Legitimization

Goals, both stated and unstated, have a way of providing their own legitimacy for an organization's or individual's activities. If a voluntary organization has a goal of providing health services to home-bound individuals, it can with great ease legitimately extend its boundaries of operation to include a gamut of activities that are not thought of as traditional health services. Perhaps the most dramatic example of this, which has already passed into the folklore of American medical care, is the work of Dr. Jack Geiger at the Mound Bayou Health Center. When he and his team arrived in that depressed area of Mississippi to set up a health center funded by the Office of Economic Opportunity, they found the social and economic problems to be considerably more pressing than the health problems. Their solution was not simply to prescribe drugs but to prescribe other necessities—most notably food. Within the context of the general goals of those programs, what Geiger and his group did was unique, but it was also within the legitimate goals of the program.

On the other hand, with no goals or only the vaguest of them, it is difficult to win support for virtually anything and even more difficult to sustain support. Simply stated, why buy a pig in a poke?

Measurement

One of the most common reasons for setting goals is measurement. Most people have been socialized from early childhood to achieve in one way or another. Growth charts, scales, reports, and myriad other sorts of documentations make it clear that some predetermined goals should be met. The underlying problem in all of this is that most people also have a natural tendency to set goals that can be measured, even though those measurable goals may have little to do with what is to be achieved. The worst example in recent American history is the body count mentality of the military during the Vietnam war. Our daily papers were filled with data on how the United States was "winning," and "winning" was defined as the number of people killed and tons of bombs dropped. The ideal of "winning hearts and minds" was somehow translated into something much more measurable. Perhaps this explains our interest, bordering on fascination, with such data as occupancy rates, average lengths of stay, and cost per day. Clearly, it is convenient to have something easily measurable.

Several years ago, these problems of measurement led this author to engage in a research project to develop a single "consumer price index" of health. The idea was to find an easily understandable measure of the changes in an individual's and a community's health status. In the sense of developing or discovering such an index, the project was a failure. What it did demonstrate were the complexities of finding a clear measure when a clear goal was equally diffuse. It is difficult indeed to measure progress toward a goal when that goal is unclear, unidentified, or controversial. An analogy might be made with a ship proceeding at great speed on a cruise to nowhere or a jet traveling eastward at 500 miles per hour with everyone (passengers, pilot, navigator, stockholders, and air controllers) disagreeing or uncertain as to where the plane should go—great progress, but to what end? In our health system, the current goal is cost containment, but how does that relate to the individual's or community's health status?

CONSTRAINTS ON HEALTH SYSTEM GOALS

A consideration of the stated and real goals of the health system is important to management, since so much of managerial behavior is related to an organization's goal. No system operates in a vacuum, however, and it must be recognized that the health system has significant constraints on its goals.

Legal Constraints

One major and increasingly important constraint is the legal one. Court-rendered definitions of health have profound operational implications; a court's interpretation of health can grant or deny jurisdiction to a health department or agency, deny or award claims for insurance and injuries, close down businesses, and enforce warranty provisions. In 1852, for example, the North Carolina Supreme Court noted in *Bell v. Jeffreys* that: "In its ordinary usage, healthy means free from disease or bodily ailment, or a state of the system peculiarly susceptible or liable to disease or bodily ailment." But the court said that when the word *sound* is added to the word *healthy* it means "whole, right, nothing the matter with it, [and] free of any defect." In this case, the plaintiff was attempting to recover damages that he had sustained through the purchase of a female slave who was supposed to be "sound and healthy" but was myopic. The nearsightedness, the plaintiff claimed, precluded the slave from performing "the common and ordinary business in the house or field, which slaves are taught and expected to perform and which is usually required of them."[12]

The issue of health again came before the North Carolina Supreme Court in 1857 when a person, after buying a slave who was warranted to be "sound in mind and body" found that the slave had a "contraction of the little finger of each hand." The contraction, the owner argued, made the slave less than healthy and justified the awarding of damages to the plaintiff. After three pages of opinion that interpreted health, healthy, and sound by quoting from a variety of regular and medical dictionaries, the court decided that, although the contracted fingers did make the slave somewhat less than useful and therefore somewhat less than healthy, the basic warrant was not broken.[13]

The modern legal definition was first stated in 1928 by the West Virginia Supreme Court of Appeals in *Venerable* v. *Gulf Taxi Line*.[14] The court said, "Health means the state of being hale, sound or whole in body, mind, soul or well-being." This legal definition is not very far removed from the North Carolina court's definitions of the 1850s or the World Health Organization's definition in the twentieth century: "Health is a state of complete physical, mental, and social well being, and not merely the absence of diseases and infirmity."[15]

Political Constraints

The political process can and does shape or even distort goals. Several years ago, state legislators in Louisiana were asked about the significance of various health status indicators on their budgetary decisions. In general, the indicators that were important to these politicians were those that are most commonly heard, although not necessarily understood, such as infant mortality rates. Perhaps of greater interest than the statistics from the study are excerpts from some of the letters from these Louisiana legislators:

I support health services with specifics—I leave this to the experts; in other words, I supply dollars. How they are parceled out and what the priorities are is not my decision to make.

Aside from local health problems with which I am familiar, the Louisiana health programs are presented to the Legislature on recommendation by the Governor. Only vague generalizations are used to support needed appropriations. Maybe the budget committee sees such statistics, but I haven't.

To be quite candid, none of these particular points [health indicators] were instrumental in making my decision and I have serious doubts that they were in the minds of practically any other member of the Legislature. In the short time we had, the entire Legislature was generally guided by the Governor's suggestions, the amount of allocations received during the past years, and on general advice from people such as Senator [X], a good friend of mine whom I personally relied upon. This is not the best way to handle these matters . . . but we have no assistance . . . and this system just does not allow for detailed study.

It is my belief that each person has the responsibility of providing the means to pay for his own health care. It seems unjust to me that the people of this State are taxed in order to pay for the health care of others. . . . I believe that the factors listed in your questionnaire . . . are the proper concern of professionals who practice in the health field and that they are not the proper concerns of politicians. State legislators have no more business trying to run the health care business than they would in trying to run the grocery business.

Professional Constraints

The role of professionals in setting goals for health care organizations cannot be minimized. To conceptualize this point, it is necessary to understand something about the ritual that physicians—the group with whom most managers have to work most closely—have passed through en route to their medical degree. This ritual of an extended educational experience, the acquisition of technical and social skills, and a value system that is the exclusive property of the profession, results in a professional philosophy that holds as almost sacrosanct the idea of autonomy— only members of the profession are qualified to evaluate or discipline other members. The loyalty of most professionals is to their profession, not to the organization for which they work. The goal orientation then is toward professional goals; in medicine, for example, these goals might be technical excellence rather than an organizational goal. Conflict comes when the profession's goals diverge from the organization's.

A case in point might be a well-insured consumer with a low back pain problem. The orthopedist examines the patient and feels that the most appropriate treatment would be ten days of complete bed rest. The physician says, "You have two choices: seven to ten days at the Community Hospital or seven to ten days at home." The patient asks, "What will happen at the hospital that couldn't occur at home?'' The physician responds, ''Essentially nothing of note—the nurses will bring you muscle relaxant medication, we'll do a few more lab tests, take a series of x-rays, and we'll know for certain that you've been on complete bed rest.'' Because of the health insurance, there will be little direct cost to the consumer for the hospitalization. There will be the costs involved in time lost from work and the costs of home care, although the latter will usually seem minimal when the family is intact. For the physician, hospitalization makes patient management more certain, since patient compliance is likely to be higher in the hospital than at home; in addition, a bill for the equivalent of one or two visits made while the patient was hospitalized would appear appropriate. In all likelihood, the hospital utilization review committee will not balk at this hospitalization, which is usually considered reasonable and conservative treatment of a common problem. For the health system, however, the costs are dramatic: seven days in the hospital at $200 per day versus seven days at home or even the Ritz with room service. It could be argued that x-rays are not available at the Ritz, but a hospitalization is hardly justified simply for x-rays or perhaps even for patient compliance. On the other hand, the health system is not set up to handle many of the "walking wounded."

In this case, the goals of the consumer and professional can easily be met by either option. In all likelihood, the decision will be made on the basis of social factors, such as attitudes about hospitalization or availability of people to care for the patient at home. The hospitalization option is extremely expensive for the health system, however, and its goal of minimizing costs is simply not considered by the two principals in the decision process: the consumer and the professional.

GOALS OF A PRISON HEALTH SYSTEM

As has been discussed, the objectives or goals of an organization are of profound importance, not only to the organization itself but also to the various constituencies it serves. The goals themselves set a legitimate direction and allow measurement of progress toward the attainment of the goal. Under the best of circumstances, objectives are clear, understandable by those who must work in the organization as well as by those outside the organization, and measurable in the sense that there is a reasonably direct way of analyzing how well the total organization is performing vis-à-vis the goals and to what extent each component is contributing toward the goal.

How this works in practice is pointedly illustrated in a consideration of the objectives of the consumers, professionals, and provider organizations in delivering health care to prison inmates. To begin with, the organization has an overriding goal of custody; no warden, sheriff, or guard is going to maintain his or her job and no prison is going to maintain its budget allocation without keeping the inmates in custody. This goal, although at first it seems obvious and indeed simplistic, is in fact crucial to an understanding of prison health problems. A second and related organizational goal is control, which translates into "keeping the place quiet." The positive goal of rehabilitation is often mentioned, but the attitude that prisons are not the place for rehabilitation but rather for punishment is becoming more prevalent. For example, in New York State there is movement toward the elimination of indeterminant sentencing. This type of sentence is designed to keep inmates in prison until they are rehabilitated, almost regardless of the length of time it takes, and it has been a significant element in the rehabilitation philosophy.

A few and often forgotten goals of prisons relate to their role in the political affairs of a community. In some instances, they are sources of political patronage jobs, although this is no longer so common; in other cases, they are led by elected officials who must be reelected or who have an interest in higher political office. From the organization's perspective then, the goals of its medical service must be related to the general organizational goals. Thus, medical care might be delayed or denied because no guard is available to escort an ailing inmate, or tranquilizers might be heavily prescribed in order to keep the prison quiet—behavior that would be considered inappropriate in a "free" health system.

Consumers also approach the health system differently inside prison, in large measure because they are forced to by circumstances. For example, a consumer in the "free world" has access to considerable medical information and a range of different opportunities and incentives with regard to the health system. "Free world" persons are encouraged to take care of themselves (to an extent) via health education programs and commercial advertisements, and pharmacies are fully stocked with over-the-counter medications that can seemingly cure anything. Rare is the house without some aspirin, Vaseline, or Band-aids. In many penal institutions, however, even these basics are denied. Thus, inmates with a headache are often required to seek medical attention simply to get what would be readily available if they were not incarcerated. Parenthetically, it should be noted that, since approximately half of the prisons in the United States do not have any medical facilities, sometimes this type of basic medical care is dispensed by the correctional staff; as has been documented in the past, staff members might dispense this care inequitably. So an inmate obtaining medical care within a prison may be attempting to attain different objectives than is a person in the outside world. An inmate, locked in a cell for a majority of the hours in a day, may want to go to the medical department simply to alleviate boredom. Who in the "free world" visits a physician out of boredom?

If the physician prescribes a medication, that medication usually has an economic value in the prison. A Valium or other tranquilizer could be sold to another inmate for money, sex, or sometimes an inmate's personal security. Most people outside of prisons do not think of visiting a physician in order to get a prescription for subsequent resale, but some consumers within penal institutions do—thus, another demand on the system.

Another set of objectives or goals from this group of consumers is escape. As noted earlier, one type is escape from boredom. There are two other types of escape: escape from work and escape from prison. Escape from work is usually conditional, based on some kind of extenuating circumstances. One of the most reasonable circumstances is an illness that precludes a person from working. In this situation, the health system plays the role of "legitimizer" of a person's health status. Thus, inmates who want to avoid a day in the laundry or at the license plate stamping machine have to convince the medical staff that they are in no condition to work. They cannot simply call in sick and have it charged to their sick leave or annual leave; they cannot simply fail to show up. It should be noted that there are some similarities to this situation in the general work force. For example, some organizations have a rule that after three days of sick leave a person must bring in a physician's note. In view of the difficulty of getting an appointment with a physician, this perhaps explains some of the emergency room crush.

A final type of escape is the classical one. While going to a prison's medical department per se does not increase an inmate's chance of escape, it might be important if it is determined that the inmate requires secondary or tertiary care in a hospital without a prison ward (and that is almost all of them). In such a situation, the inmate is usually guarded by a security staff; within the confines of a hospital, however, there are few backup security systems or even an attitude that is custody-oriented. Thus, a determined inmate, particularly with help from friends, would have a much simpler time escaping from a hospital than from a penal institution. But the medical department sits in judgment about who shall go to the hospital and who shall receive treatment inside the walls.

The difficulty of coordinating these goals in practice can be seen in the case of an aged, acutely ill patient who was delayed in a county jail about 30 minutes while a security crew was rounded up for this almost comatose patient. Clearly, the custody goal reigned supreme over the care goals.

The third group of goals in this example are those of the professionals: the physicians, nurses, and paraprofessionals who deliver the care. Their primary professional goal is the provision of high quality clinical care in an efficient and effective manner. However, the prison health system also requires them to be traffic cops and triage the sick from the malingerers. It also asks them to utilize their skills to assist in the custodial functions: "be liberal with the tranquilizers; it's better to have a bunch of quiet zonked inmates than anxious obstreperous ones." While this might be less than optimum medical care, it is effective "wardening." Thus, the medical department is, for the most part through no fault of its own, placed in a most uncomfortable position. It knows what it wants to do, but the demands made by the organization and consumer require behavior that, while unpleasant and at the margins of professional acceptability, is quite clearly necessary for survival.

Finally, constraining all of this is a host of political variables, such as the political ambitions of sheriffs or mayors, the economic realities of government (this is one area the free enterprise system has avoided), and philosophies; for example, does the country at large really care about those persons who are incarcerated? Since most people do not consider themselves vulnerable on that account, they can easily avoid this issue in their complicated lives.

In the private sector, it is often heard that goals boil down to the "bottom line," but translating this into an operational objective becomes difficult. It is appropriate to close this chapter by recounting Lynn Townsend's experience at AVIS, where it took six months for his firm to come up with its business objective of "renting and leasing vehicles without drivers."[16] The delineation and acceptance of this goal had profound implications; it caused AVIS to get or stay out of the hotel business, tour bus business, and so forth. As AVIS and others have learned, clear goals and objectives are hard to come by, but once obtained they allow a concentration of effort that results in a more efficient and effective organization.

CASE STUDY

The Orleans Parish Prison Case

Author's Note: This case is presented for illustrative purposes. A detailed discussion of other dimensions of this case and related matters can be found in an earlier book by the author, *Prison Health* (New York: Prodist, 1975). Also, it should be noted that, thanks to the efforts of the federal court, its appointed Special Master, the criminal sheriffs, and numerous others, the medical care situation at Orleans Parish Prison has improved dramatically since this case study was originally prepared.

During the fall of 1969, a group of inmates at Orleans Parish Prison filed a class action suit in the U.S. Federal District Court of Louisiana against the mayor of New Orleans, the city council representatives, the Orleans Parish Criminal Sheriff, and the prison's warden. The inmates charged that they had been systematically deprived of their rights under the Eighth Amendment to the Constitution in that conditions at the Orleans Parish Prison were such as to constitute cruel and inhuman punishment.

The following were the federal judges' major findings of fact relative to health care at the facility:

The danger of an outbreak of contagious diseases is great as a result of the unsanitary conditions in the toilets, the kitchen and sleeping equipment. Further, no medical intake survey is made to detect prisoners with contagious diseases. Although the incidence of gonorrhea is high, only sporadic blood tests for syphilis are done. As a result of the crowded conditions, there is no isolation or quarantine area for those with contagious diseases that are detected.

The combined effects of the fearful atmosphere and crowded and sordid living conditions has a severe effect on psychotics, often causing those transferred to the prison from mental hospitals. Disruptive psychotic prisoners are sometimes moved into a hallway by the main gate and shackled to the bars.

Hospital facilities and medical attention are woefully inadequate to meet the needs of the inmates. Inmates who should be confined to bed with chronic diseases must be kept on the open tiers. Medication that is prescribed frequently never reaches the inmate or else is taken from him by other prisoners.[17]

The key individuals involved in the lawsuit and their relationship to the prison were the following:

- inmates: prisoners within jail
- mayor: popularly elected official serving a four-year term; full-time responsibility
- city council: elected officials; most city councilmen had outside employment
- criminal sheriff: elected official with part-time law practice
- warden: full-time civil service appointed position
- prison doctor: originally, a full-time position; now part-time at minimal compensation; theoretically on-call, but rarely called
- nurse: full-time, 40 hours per week civil service appointment
- pharmacist: budgeted for full-time working 10-15 hours per week; civil service appointment

The prison is organized in a bureaucratic manner with the criminal sheriff as the chief executive officer and the warden as his primary deputy. The prison doctor, pharmacist, and nurse report to the warden and sheriff. The total budget for the program, which serviced approximately 800 inmates, was $69,000 per year. The quality of care delivered under this system was poor.

After an extensive investigation, it was recommended that Orleans Parish Prison enter into a specific performance contract with an appropriately qualified medical group to deliver medical services to Orleans Parish prisoners. Under this plan, administrative authority should be retained by the criminal sheriff; professional responsibility should be placed in the hands of the contracting group; and the City of New Orleans Health Department should be given responsibility for monitoring the quality of medical care provided. Basically, the contractor should agree to perform routine intake physical examinations and conduct routine sick call for all inmates on a 24-hour basis. Additionally, the contractor should agree to provide comprehensive backup consultative services—medical, surgical, obstetrical, and psychiatric—as well as emergency medical services; medications were to be ordered on a cost basis. The contractee (the Orleans Parish Prison and the City of New Orleans) should agree to provide appropriate physical space, equipment, and supplies and to reimburse the contractor for services of medical and nonmedical personnel and supplies.

The changes as recommended represented a new budget of $138,000 per year, 50 hours of physician time per week, and complete laboratory workups for inmates.

Discussion Questions

1. What objections are likely to be raised to the proposed program by the key individuals in the case?
2. What are likely to be the obstacles to the implementation of such a plan?

NOTES

1. G.A. Theodorson, and A.G. Theodorson, *Modern Dictionary of Sociology* (New York: Cromwell, 1969), p. 431.
2. C.W. Churchman, *The Systems Approach* (New York: Delacorte Press, 1968), p. 29.
3. R.A. Johnson, F.E. Kast, and J.E. Rosenzweig, *The Theory and Management of Systems*, 2nd ed. (New York: McGraw-Hill, 1967), p. 4.
4. American Public Health Association, *A Guide to Medical Care Administration* Vol. I, *Concepts and Principles*, 1964, p. 15.
5. I.M. Rosenstock, "Why People Use Health Services," *Milbank Memorial Fund Quarterly*, XLIV, no. 3 (July 1966): 94-124.
6. S.W. Bloom, *The Doctor and His Patient* (New York: Free Press, 1963), 1965.
7. M. Shain, and M. Roemer, "Hospital Costs Relate to Supply of Beds," *Modern Hospital* 92 (April 1959): 71.
8. A. Jacobi, "The Best Means of Combating Infant Mortality," *Journal of the American Medical Association*, 58, no. 23 (June 8, 1912): 1735-1744.
9. F.E. Korbin, "The American Midwife Controversy: A Crisis of Professionalization," *Bulletin of the History of Medicine* XL, no. 4 (July-August 1966): 350-363.
10. S.B. Goldsmith, "House Calls: Anachronism or Advent," *Public Health Reports* 94, no. 4 (July-August 1979): 299-304.

11. For a more detailed discussion and analysis of prison health, see L.F. Novick, and M.S. Al-Ibrahim, *Health Problems in the Prison Setting* (Springfield, IL: Charles C. Thomas, 1977) and S.B. Goldsmith, *Prison Health* (New York: Prodist, 1975).

12. *Bell v. Jeffreys,* 35 N.C. 356 (1852).

13. *Harrell v. Norvill,* 50 N.C. 29 (1857).

14. *Venerable v. Gulf Taxi Line,* 141 S.E. 622 (1928).

15. World Health Organization: The first ten years of the World Health Organization, WHO, Geneva, 1958, p. 459.

16. R. Townsend, *Up the Organization* (Greenwich, CT: Fawcett, 1970), pp. 111-112.

17. *Louis Hamilton et al.* v. *Victor Shiro et al.,* U.S. Dist. Ct., Eastern Dist., La., New Orleans Div., Case No. 69-2443, pp. 3-5.

Chapter 5

Management in Industry and Health Care

Virtually every textbook dealing with management at some point offers the reader a definition of the subject. For example, in 1947 Cornell answered the question, What is management, by noting

> The work of management is to plan, direct and control the organization and to weave together its various parts so that all factors will function properly and all persons cooperate—that is, work together efficiently— for a common purpose.[1]

Gibson, Ivancevich, and Donnelly, in their popular text, note that "management is a set of activities which can be classified as concerned with planning, organizing or controlling."[2] In perhaps one of the grandest understatements, Drucker, in his best-selling book *Management,* suggests that "management is tasks, discipline, people and practice."[3] Management must be viewed as both an art and a science. On one hand, it deals with sharply defined areas, such as productivity and efficiency, that are exemplified best in current times by the operations, research/ management science approach to problem solving. On the other hand, it also deals in more diffuse areas, such as leadership and motivation.

For the manager, this sets up a challenge. How does the manager construct or reconstruct organizations so that they maximize efficiency and effectiveness to their various external constituencies and simultaneously minimize stress, disaffection, and unhappiness to their internal constituencies? It should be recognized that this problem or challenge is a value-laden statement, as are most definitions of management and concepts of the manager's role. The emphasis in this statement is on satisfying external constituencies, performing efficiently in economic and financial terms, being effective, and, finally, respecting the human dignity of workers. If, for example, workers are considered drones, peasants, or simply inputs for a resource system, this challenge might be restated to eliminate concern with the disaffected workers. Indeed, the manager's concept of the meaning of work can very dramatically shift his or her perspective.

A management approach based on a value system, as they all are to some degree, must examine that system if it is to be responsive and continue to function as a mechanism of achieving organizational goals.

THE FUNCTIONS OF MANAGEMENT

The specific activity a manager may be involved in is likely to vary from one organization to another, as well as from time to time in the same organization. The sum total of management in an organization tends to be relatively stable, however; the same managerial functions are carried out, although circumstances, organizational needs, and personalities dictate which of these functions predominates at any given time. The most often cited of these functions are planning, organizing, staffing, directing, controlling, coordinating, and representing.

Planning

Planning involves those activities associated with objective setting, policy making, and strategies for attaining objectives within the organizational policy framework. As noted earlier, it is considerably more difficult to identify objectives, particularly in the health field, than it appears at first glance. Organizational objective setting is a process that requires global vision, diplomatic skill, and considerable good fortune. Planning normally results in an output; that is, a written plan. Such a document can cover periods of time that vary from rather short periods, such as six months or a year, to five or ten years. An effective plan results in a positive outcome for the organization; a bad plan is likely to be worse than no plan because of the tendency to honor the written word.

Individuals who serve as planners in organizations may seem to take that responsibility off the shoulders of management, but this is an illusion. Management never totally delegates this responsibility or authority. A plan is the organizational control device. With a plan, management can continually identify expectations (goals) for people, programs, or projects and measure the progress and the rate of progress being made toward these goals. Some managers prefer to utilize the lack of a plan as a control device for their organizations; the only plan is what is in the manager's head. In this way, the manager maintains total control and great flexibility but reigns over a situation that may often be close to disaster.

In the health field, particularly hospitals, planning is viewed as both necessary and positive. It is necessary as a result of external factors, such as the fact that Health Systems Agencies (HSAs) require one- or five-year plans; it is positive simply because many organizations have found that strategic planning has been in their best interest.

Organizing

Organizing is a second function commonly associated with management. This is the function of determining what activities shall be carried out in the organization, how these activities should be grouped, and who shall have the authority and responsibility for carrying out these activities. The control device for this function is the organizational structure. In practical terms, this may explain why some organizations seem to be in a continual state of reorganization—managers are trying to gain control through this managerial function.

There are considerable constraints, however, on the value of the organizing function and the manager's use of it. For example, a new organization chart on which mediocre staff members are shifted to new "boxes" may simply be an illusion of progress. Occasionally, such a shakeup has a positive effect—but in the health field, where a significant number of people are in the public sector (government of one level or another), change through reorganization may be viewed as another temporary and feeble attempt of management to control the organization. One cannot help but wonder whether all the changes at the U.S. Department of Health and Human Services (HHS) have done more than generate enormous confusion, countless office changes, and power exercise for senior administrators. Has there been any substantive program change that could not have been accomplished without the reorganization?

In the health field, legal and fiscal constraints, such as third party reimbursement requirements, dictate certain elements of organizational structure. Tradition and the reality of staffing generate other structural requirements. Could pathologists be recruited if the organizational structure were such that they reported to a nonphysician laboratory manager? The conflict engendered by having registered nurses report to nonphysician, nonnurse ward managers must also be considered. Professionalism of all types is deeply ingrained in the health field and is a force to be reckoned with in the organizing function.

Staffing

Staffing is perhaps the most obvious, most useful, and most critical of management functions. Basically, this involves getting the right people for the jobs and developing them. Theoretical control devices for this function are personnel management tools, such as job descriptions, job specifications, and, of course, the budget. The exercise of these control devices might be illustrated by three examples from the world of academia. In one instance, a new university president was hired, and he made his first priority that of building a high quality faculty, a difficult task in a university with more than its share of marginal faculty. His strategy was to use the management functions of staffing and budget; he personally reviewed every candidate for a faculty position and refused to sign the papers authorizing the hiring of anyone who did not meet his standards.

In a different university, with an equally marginal faculty, it was decided to build a new department. Two options were presented: (a) draw faculty from related departments or (b) acquire a whole new staff for the department. Although option (a) was quite attractive because it could cut the time frame from inception to optimal operation by years—perhaps a decade—it also represented a commitment to the qualitative status quo. Option (b) was selected, and within ten years the new department became the leader in its field, despite the overall reputation of the university.

A final example involves a distinguished university that was awarded a one-time grant of $2 million to start a research center. Here again, two options were considered: (a) spend the money to attract a limited number of senior researchers and hope their work would generate funds in the future to keep the operation viable, or (b) build a high quality support system of junior staff, such as research assistants and secretaries, and hardware, such as computers, and hope that some of these people develop into researchers able to generate funds and/or that the support systems attract the senior researchers. In this case option (b) was selected. Within five years, no senior researchers had been attracted, the junior researchers had produced little, and the research center was forced out of business.

These illustrations point up the critical nature of the staffing function in management. Staff make or break an organization, and people develop other people. Although a resource-consuming and often discouraging activity, staffing either will bring healthy blood into an organization or will create a potentially debilitating influence.

It is interesting to consider how often industry utilizes "headhunters" and how reluctant health care organizations are to undertake careful executive searches. For example, in one hospital, a young physician was hired as a full-time employee at a salary in excess of $40,000 after a 30-minute interview with no checking of credentials, recommendations, or "second opinions."

Directing

Directing is the function most often associated with management. Many people view managers as sitting in their offices, no doubt quite removed from any part of the operation, and barking out orders to a compliant group of employees. Except in rare cases, this is a fantasy. Managers may like to view themselves as captains of ships, but their word is no longer the law. Rather, they must use their position to guide, persuade, or coach subordinates. The control device is less the organizational position than the ability to lead and motivate. Even in highly bureaucratic organizations, such as universities or hospitals, management is by consensus, and the effective manager must shepherd that consensus to meet goals.

Health care managers should always remember that few physicians, no matter how low they are on the organizational totem pole, ever walk into the director's office and think they are going to the "boss."

Controlling

Controlling, a fifth function, is concerned with the measurement of performance against some predetermined standard. Two elements must come together if the manager's control is going to be effective: (a) there must be standards; and (b) there must be information systems to indicate the progress that is being made toward attaining those standards.

One example of an effective control device is the budget and its companion budgeting process. For example, an organization may have a clear budgeting process that not only projects revenues and expenses but also requires targets and reviews. In accepting a given department's budget and holding it accountable for its projections, the manager is controlling the department's activities. If ambulatory care projected expenses of $1 million for the fiscal year and seven-eighths of the way through the year came to the manager with a request for more money to hire a new staff person, the manager can now use the controlling function via the budget to direct the organization. Money and ego are probably two of the most potent controlling mechanisms—ego being the more difficult to deal with since there are few "performance standards" and information systems about egos are limited, at best.

Coordinating

Coordinating is a sixth function and, in some senses, one of the weakest. Traditionally, a coordinator has plenty of responsibility and little authority—analogous to the carpenter who is given wood and nails but no hammer. It appears that the most successful coordinators are those with real or apparent authority, a total commitment to the program, or extraordinary skills as a persuader. To put it differently, important managerial problems are too complex both in terms of the problem itself and the system that has generated the problem to be "coordinated." They must be "managed" in an affirmative manner.

Representing

The seventh traditional function is representing or being the spokesman for the unit, organization, or industry on the outside. A department head represents the department and its case on the division level, and the director represents the organization to the government, a foundation, or even the board.

Representation is a critical managerial function. Those on top of each component usually represent the component to those on the next higher level. This is a time- and energy-consuming function that requires a political sensitivity to the needs of a constituency (or unit) and a similar sensitivity to the needs of those to whom the constituency is being represented. The skills of presentation, debate, analysis, and articulation are critical, since they are weighed in the minds of those who are listening to the presentation.

Developing People

A slightly different view is presented by Drucker, whose perspective is that the management role has four basic elements: (1) objective setting, (2) organization, (3) measurement, and (4) developing people. This last element is perhaps the most critical and the one usually not identified by other writers in the field.[4] Developing people suggests a high level of commitment to the maximal utilization of human resources, which becomes critical in a labor-intensive industry such as health care. Obviously, in the health field, there are constraints because of the technical dimensions of many jobs and the concomitant legal constraints.

WHO IS A MANAGER?

A traditionist would say "anyone who gets things done through other people is a manager," which portrays the manager as the grand puppeteer. Perhaps a less offensive approach might be to say that a manager is anyone who is not personally involved in the direct implementation of the work. A manager then is someone who is involved in a range of activities, but a manager's responsibility stops short of personal implementation of these activities. A manager might be someone involved in creating an innovative ambulatory care program, putting it together so that it becomes a reality, or evaluating it for further nurturing or retrenching.

Particularly in health care, it seems that managers expend a great deal of their time fighting "forest fires"—chasing a solution for small problems. These problems are part of a larger system and context, a point often overlooked in dealing with the specific fire.

In general, managers can be classified into two groups: staff and line. In contrast to the staff or supportive function manager, the line manager is generally thought to be directly involved in the production functions of the organization. The line of distinction is blurred, however, when certain functions are discussed as line and others as staff. For example, personnel departments are usually regarded as staff—but what about the personnel manager who has 35 employees reporting to him?

As a generality (which is certainly open to challenge), line managers appear to thrive when dealing with action-oriented problems. Scores of telephone calls and appointments seem to fan the fire of their systems. On the other hand, staff managers appear to be more deliberative, attempt to analyze all the angles, and, in the words of one executive "headhunter," take fewer risks.

Line managers are sometimes criticized for "shooting from the hip"—a charge that may be based on form rather than substance. Rapid information processing based on experience and expertise often appears to be "hip shooting" but may in fact be effective management. Indeed, it is an example of the critical information-processing thread that is common to all the activities of management. Managers must transmit, receive, and interpret verbal, nonverbal, and written information.

The transmission mechanisms include one-to-one and one-to-group communications, memos, newsletters, press releases, letters, facial expressions, tones of voice, selected words, and others. By choice of the medium and method of delivery, the manager is making a statement, such as "I am the boss," "Let's share as equals," or "Your work or being means nothing to me." As a recipient of information, a similar process occurs in reverse.

Interpretation of information received is probably one of the most critical activities associated with processing. "What did that memo mean?" An effective manager does not simply react to what is said but rather attempts to understand what is meant by what is said. Such skill in communication can be developed and is invaluable to a manager.

EXPECTATIONS FROM MANAGERS

What should be expected from a manager? In answering this question, two dimensions must be considered: behavior and values

Both fiction and reality have presented a picture of managers as "organization men." Their loyalty is with the organization, and the most important professional person in their lives is their boss. The image (and reality, to a great extent) is of a tight hierarchical structure and operations that respond to that structure. Regardless of the theoretical "flatness" of the organization, there is always someone on the top who has the authority and responsibility to represent the organization and negotiate for its well-being—at least that person's concept of its well-being.

A clear example of this is the case of the attempted takeover of McGraw-Hill by American Express. This takeover was viewed as an anathema by McGraw-Hill's chairman, Harold McGraw, Jr. Because of his personal view, he waged a relentless and successful campaign against the invasion. He stated in a letter to the chief executive officer of American Express that American Express lacked "integrity, corporate morality and sensitivity to professional responsibility."[5] He went on to criticize the management and behavior of American Express. All of this was carried out with the express approval of stockholders, many of whom clearly stood to gain by such a merger.

A different perspective on management is presented by Michael Blumenthal. During his tenure as secretary of the Treasury, he prepared an article for *Fortune* titled "Candid Reflections of a Businessman in Washington."[6] In it, he contrasted his experiences as a senior government official in charge of an agency employing 120,000 people with his position as chairman and chief executive officer of the Bendix Corporation. Control, he suggests, is related to the ability to "hire and fire"—he identified his problem in government: "Out of 120,000 people in the Treasury, I was able to select twenty-five maybe. The other 119,975 are outside my control."

It was noted earlier that top management is involved in goal setting and organizing activities that allow the goals to be attained. The contrast between the private and public sectors was highlighted when Blumenthal noted that the senior executives in industry can control who is and is not involved in policy development and implementation; but because of the plethora of official and nonofficial interest groups in government, many of whom have influence and power, the policy process is considerably more complex.

A final point is that management in industry does most of its business in private. Government executives, however, must function under the spotlight of the press.

How then do the expectations of the health care manager differ from those of the industrial manager? In a newspaper article about the recipient of the American College of Hospital Administrators "Young Hospital Administrator of the Year Award," it was pointed out that the award winner had "superior administrative capability," which was demonstrated in a variety of ways, including the quality of care at the institution, the physical and programmatic growth of the hospital, the financial health of the hospital, and its positive professional image. As if that were not enough, the article continued with a description of his activities as a local and national leader and ended with a statement regarding his "positive spirit." An analysis of this article suggests that, to be successful, at least in the eyes of one professional organization, people must be joiners and innovators, accept the organization's goals as their own, and invest their spiritual and physical energy in building an organization.

Two dimensions that are no doubt of the greatest importance in management are technical skills and the ability to recruit and retain able subordinates. Technical skills are oftentimes underemphasized, but they are a major element in a manager's credibility and value to an organization. For example, can the manager accurately forecast the utilization of services, and is that forecast based on a high quality assessment of needs, likely demands, and competition? Can the manager develop an appropriate strategic plan or budget for the organization? This does not mean that the manager must write the budget personally, but he or she must plan, organize, and review the budget before it is placed in the hands of the board. Mistakes, conceptual or mechanical, indicate a careless or technically unskilled manager—particularly at the beginning of a career.

If there is one shortcoming of new managers it may be an overreliance on the importance of their image as managers and an underreliance on the technical substance that is expected from them.

Since few managers, even workaholics, have the time and ability to do everything themselves, they must rely on subordinates for their own success. Managers' ability to find people who will be supportive and complement their own skills is crucial. Some managers view high quality subordinates as threats and hire sycophants. Others view them as tools to carry out unpleasant jobs and hire "hatchet men." A third group view subordinates as key colleagues, and they attempt to surround themselves with the best people available. One problem with the "best and brightest" is that they tend to move on if new challenges are not forthcoming, however.

The organizational environment has a personal impact on the manager. One organization may be very private and look for individuals who conduct themselves in a reserved manner. An aggressive organization may seek a different personality type. Several years ago, in a study of Geisinger Medical Center, it was noted that when staff members (presumably male) were recruited, the spouses and children were also interviewed in order to make sure that the family was the "right" type. Geisinger was attempting to ensure that the people recruited understood and could personally thrive in an unusual rural community while contributing professionally to an outstanding and somewhat unique group practice and hospital. Some people reacted negatively to this practice, feeling that Geisinger's behavior was offensive and beyond the borders of appropriate recruiting protocol. In fact, this policy is not dissimilar from that of many large corporations and, within the context of their goals, problems, and experience, it makes a great deal of sense. As the British have noted many times before, however, "It is not everyone's cup of tea."

VALUES AND ETHICS IN MANAGEMENT

In the rush of managerial firefighting, it is often forgotten that much decision making is preprogrammed by something akin to an inertial guidance system that is directed by the decision maker's value orientation. This value orientation is a complex set of beliefs and attitudes that eventually manifest themselves in behavior. Guth and Tagiuri, using a general value scale conceptualized by Spanger, studied corporate executives and found that their orientation was highest in the direction of "economic man," "theoretical man," and "political man;" lowest in terms of value orientations that characterized "religious man," "aesthetic man," and "social man."[7]

The following definitions were used by Guth and Tagiuri for their value orientation terms:

- The "theoretical man" is primarily interested in the discovery of truth, in the systematic ordering of his knowledge. In pursuing this goal he typically takes a "cognitive" approach, looking for identities and differences, with relative disregard for the beauty or utility of objects, seeking only to observe and to reason. His interests are empirical, critical, and rational. He is an intellectual. Scientists or philosophers are often of this type.

• The "economic man" is primarily oriented toward what is useful. He is interested in the practical affairs of the business world; in the production, marketing, and consumption of goods; in the use of economic resources; and in the accumulation of tangible wealth. He is thoroughly "practical" and fits well the stereotype of the American businessman.

• The "aesthetic man" finds his chief interest in the artistic aspects of life, although he need not be a creative artist. He values form and harmony. He views experience in terms of grace, symmetry, or harmony. Each single event is savored for its own sake.

• The essential value for the "social man" is love of people—the altruistic or philanthropic aspect of love. The social man values people as ends, and tends to be kind, sympathetic, and unselfish. He finds those who have strong theoretical, economic, and aesthetic orientations rather cold. Unlike the political type, the social man regards love as the most important component of human relationships. In its purest form the social orientation is selfless and approaches the religious attitude.

• The "political man" is characteristically oriented toward power, not necessarily in politics, but in whatever area he functions. Most leaders have a high power orientation. Competition plays a large role in all life, and many writers have regarded power as the most universal motive. For some men, this motive is uppermost, driving them to seek personal power, influence, and recognition.

• The "religious man" is one "whose mental structure is permanently directed to the creation of the highest and absolutely satisfying value experience." The dominant value for him is unity. He seeks to relate himself to the universe in a meaningful way and has a mystical orientation.

A few years ago, a group of first year graduate students in health administration were asked to rank on a scale of 1 to 5 various types of managers, based on the students' perception of the value orientation of these managers. The students' views (Table 5-1) were similar to that of Guth and Tagiuri for industrial managers. They believed that typical health care and hospital managers share the value system of other managers, and they viewed themselves as also sharing the value system, but without the intensity of the others. In general, they also had a perceived low value for religious, aesthetic, and social orientations among managers, although they viewed themselves as socially oriented. This demonstrates one

Table 5-1 Ranking of Value Orientation of Various Managers

	Mean Rankings		
	Industrial Manager	Health Care Manager	Hospital Administrator
Theoretical	3.6	3.3	3.1
Economic	1.28	2.6	1.6
Aesthetic	4.7	5.09	5.09
Social	4.47	3.42	4.0
Political	2.09	2.71	2.6
Religious	4.5	5.81	5.3

Source: Reprinted by permission of the Harvard Business Review. Exhibit from "Personal Values and Corporate Strategy" by William D. Guth and Renato Tagiuri (September-October 1975). Copyright © 1975 by the President and Fellows of Harvard College; all rights reserved.

of the critical personal dilemmas in health administration: on one hand, there is the social orientation of health; on the other, the economic orientation of administration.

One distressing example of this dilemma is in the issue of ethics, more specifically ethical problems in health administration. Within the past few years a dean of a school of public health was forced to resign after he was indicted (and subsequently convicted) by a federal court of conspiracy to defraud the government; a nationally prominent hospital administrator lost his job when his organization discovered that he was double billing for his travel; a professor and chairman of a department of health administration lost his job and ended up in jail after serious wrongdoings were discerned; and seemingly countless nursing home administrators have been indicted and prosecuted for a range of offenses. These, plus numerous other examples, suggest several hypotheses regarding the ethics of health administrators: the pressure on health administrators is getting so great that the ethical fiber is breaking down at an increasing rate; the low level ethics of health administrators is finally being discovered and exposed; or, perhaps, health administrators are simply devoid of any sense of ethics.

The literature on ethics in health administration is, at best, limited. Most articles focus on the ethical and legal problems plaguing health systems or hospitals, not the administrators per se. One notable exception is Hahn's recent review titled "Ethical Conduct of the CEO."[8] In this article, the author considers the various conceptual and ethical problems facing chief executive officers. A valuable contribution is a report of a survey of course content in ethics from 28 graduate programs in health administration. Hahn found that "most programs integrate the concept of ethics in other lecture and seminar courses." This may mean that the concept is so important as to be included everywhere—or, alternatively, it is so unimportant and/or difficult to handle as to be included nowhere.

Since the available literature is often at odds with the operational reality, a special study was undertaken of the ethical problems facing three different groups of health administrators. All three groups were asked the same four questions:

1. What was the most difficult ethical decision you had to make in the past year?
2. What did you see as the major alternative decisions that could have been made?
3. What was your decision?
4. What do you see as the major implications of your decision?

Clearly, such open-ended questions were not developed to give definitive answers to the problems plaguing health administrators, but rather to set some realistic parameters on the type of ethical issues they face.

Forty-two responses from four different groups of administrators were analyzed: 12 hospital administrators, 12 drug program administrators, 10 nursing home administrators, and 8 nursing home administrators who were department heads at long-term care facilities. Of the 12 hospital administrators, 6 were chief executives and 6 were at associate levels. Although all 12 administrators were associated with similar institutions in somewhat similar communities, no two problems identified by the administrators were similar. However 5 of the 6 chief operating executives identified problems that could be classified as medical staff problems:

- oppose facility expansion desired by medical staff

- oppose employment of new physician who was needed but whose recommendations were less than satisfactory

- oppose the medical staff's position on malpractice

- integrate (racially) medical staff and trustees

- fire a senior level physician

- shorten utilization

The sixth problem, shortening utilization, had profound implications for the hospital's income and, potentially, for the individual physician's income.

Associate administrator level respondents, not surprisingly in view of the scope of their responsibility, tended to identify problems that were more operationally oriented:

- accept part-time self-serving position with potential purveyor

- support chief operating executive when personal position was contrary

- terminate a nonprofessional employee with cause but without due process

- become a "_____" complainant against a medical staff member

- reprimand medical staff

Even the reprimanding of a physician was viewed as an ethical problem. The associate director felt that the physician deserved a reprimand, but it clearly was not the decision of the hospital's board, trustees, or administration that this physician be reprimanded.

The alternatives in most instances were black and white—either do it or do not do it. In the 12 cases reviewed, the administrators found some compromise position in three instances, did what they felt they should do in seven instances, and in the remaining two cases they did or allowed something to occur that they did not support.

The second group surveyed were 18 nursing home administrators: 10 individuals in line administration who held positions such as administrator or assistant administrator and 8 persons who were in department or other supportive roles, such as social workers or dietitians.

The decision list generated by the line administrators is heavily weighted in the area of what might be classified as basic personnel management:

- order staff to come to work on time

- fire a mentally retarded worker

- reassign a team of workers

- evaluate a nurse's work

- allow an employee to leave work one-half hour early

- fire a poor quality employee

- hire an employee of another faith for a religious nursing home

- resign from a facility that is violating the law

- accept a more difficult job

- accept employment in a field (nursing home administration) that was tainted

A review of the problems identified by this group does not suggest that any momentous issues were considered. For example, one assistant administrator wrote the following:

An employee, RN, came to me last week and asked if she could take off from work ½ hour earlier because her son was going to sing in a church choir and she wanted to be with him. I decided that I would let her go with ½ hour docked off her pay.

Three of the problems were seemingly highly personal in that they involved the administrators' future. Two of those responses suggest that the authors actually went through some sort of personal crisis or soul-searching:

- Should I stay, leave, or "try to convince top management of reasons why the organization should eliminate violations?"
- Am I jeopardizing "my reputation as an upstanding citizen" by entering this field?

Although the third response was a job change decision, no ethical considerations were evident.

The staff and department administrators in nursing homes presented a range of problems that were generally dissimilar from those seen with the other administrators:

- advocate a patient's position that is in opposition to the institution's position
- voice concern about a suspicious patient injury
- investigate a patient's complaint about inadequate medications
- place Christmas trees on all floors of a kosher, nonsectarian nursing home
- maintain state health code standards
- expose serious operating deficiencies in another department
- create a harmonious work environment for staff
- enter into a relationship between a nonprofit and for-profit organization

Three of these problems were patient-oriented; two were almost classic conflict-of-interest situations; and the remaining three were general organizational problems. Perhaps this can be explained by the fact that, while many of these people see themselves as administrators, they usually function as social workers or dietitians. These are roles that are traditionally quite close physically and spiritually to patients.

The final 12 respondents were administrators of drug programs, all of whom had a background in social work and were employed in operational programs that involved the treatment of drug addicts on both an inpatient and outpatient basis. The range of problems that they identified were predominantly staff personnel matters or general policy matters:

- start termination action against a chronically ill employee
- act in a consistent manner with regard to personnel policies of time, attendance, etc.
- release an employee because of age
- hire staff primarily because of their ethnic background
- select employees for layoff
- transfer to a better job in another department with a different philosophy
- debate an administrative edict
- implement a personally unacceptable course of action
- implement a patient treatment plan that was unacceptable to the next higher level of management
- cooperate with a state investigating group

Rather surprisingly, there were few patient-oriented problems. For example, four administrators identified a hiring/firing problem as their most difficult ethical decision of the past year, and two of the three patient-related problems were general and related to a specific patient, such as the issue of whether an administrator should cooperate with a state investigating group.

This modest study suggests that administrators have few serious ethical problems. Could this be the case? This author would argue that they simply do not know what an ethical problem is. Perhaps this explanation is too harsh or too simplistic, but it should be obvious that a significant percentage of "ethical" problems identified were fairly typical administrative problems—usually involving personnel management. It appears that the broader issues of conflicts between personal values or organizational values are simply not being identified by top health care management. Perhaps this is because administrators have lulled themselves into believing that the administrative decision process is value-free—it is not, however, and it is imperative that these values be identified and analyzed. Obviously, this is not yet taking place.

ENTERING MANAGEMENT

In his text *Management,* Drucker identifies six common mistakes in designing managerial jobs. These mistakes are (1) designing "the job so small that a good man cannot grow;" (2) having a job that is not really a job; (3) having a job that does not combine work with managing; (4) having jobs that require "continuous meetings, continuous cooperation and coordination;'' (5) giving out titles rather than jobs; and (6) creating "widow-maker" jobs, that is, those that are simply impossible to do.[9] Drucker's presentation is particularly useful for a chief executive officer who must establish or reorganize an organization. However, his statements are also useful for a manager who must decide whether to accept a new position. So with apologies and acknowledgment to Drucker, the following is a list of six ideas to consider when entering or shifting positions on the managerial ladder.

Take a job in which you can grow. In the field of health administration, growth is both a function of the job and the organization. Hospitals were once the fast track for new managers; however, because of decreasing facilities, increased numbers of graduates of health administration programs, and economic controls, hospitals have become a much slower and more slippery track. Organizations that did not exist a decade ago, such as Professional Standards Review Organizations (PSROs) and HSAs, represent new opportunities for growth in the health care market. Nursing homes and ambulatory care programs, which at one time were viewed as stepchildren areas for employment, have now moved to the forefront as career opportunities.

Do not be a "go-for" for another person. Nonjobs are particularly common in the health industry and are well described by Drucker as those positions in which the title is "assistant to." An individual's performance should be observable by the total organization, and the position should not be dependent on the good will of one person. In small health care organizations, particularly at the entry levels, this is a difficult pitfall to avoid. Some managers attempt to avoid this by continually defining and redefining their positions in writing (via a series of memos). If there is good will and if those higher in the organization feel secure, there are few problems with this method. If the junior manager is simply another tool in the senior manager's bag, all the memos in the organization are insignificant compared with the opinion of the "boss." To the extent possible, then, the job should represent a commitment from the organization, not from a single person at the next level up in the chain of command.

Take a job in which you work and manage. No one can suggest that management is not hard work, but quite clearly there is a tendency for young managers to ensconce themselves in pleasant offices and deal only with those who seek them out, respond to those higher on the hierarchy, and "play the manager role." Periodically, however, managers should get their hands dirty. For the physician-manager, this is easily translated into seeing patients occasionally. For the non-physician-manager it may mean such things as handling special projects or observing certain operations. Managers must continue to develop their own competencies and periodically test these competencies by "working." Such tests and development have positive effects both in personal self-esteem and in respect from colleagues and subordinates. An analogy with academia might clarify this concept further—a dean should not only administer the school but should also work by teaching and personally doing research.

Avoid a position with a great deal of nonproductive time. Most people are measured by their output or the outcome of what they do, not the process used to attain these goals. While process is critical to reach goals, it is easy to forget that the process is not, in fact, the outcome. For example, meetings become more important than the decisions and the implementation of the decisions reached at the meetings. All positions have some of this nonproductive time, but new managers must look for positions in which this is either minimized or at least they have some control over it. Many new managers have looked back over the first few years of their jobs and found that they have spent most of their time in meetings and have been doing little. The organization in its evaluation wants the bases touched but also wants the runs scored.

Get your objectives straight–What do you really want? This is extremely difficult, because there is a strong current impelling managers toward accepting the objectives of the organization as their own. Soul-searching is often a tiring and time-consuming process, but it is a necessary one if managers are to understand what they really want from their position. Is it power, prestige, security, glamour, intellectual stimulation, money, or a combination of these and other factors? A person who has come to grips with these personal objectives is in a much stronger position to make career choices. Without addressing these personal objectives (which may be subconscious), managers may generate unnecessary and possibly debilitating anxiety in their lives.

When in doubt, maximize your potential for success by taking proven jobs. Managers should not risk their future on Drucker's widow-maker job, a job that others have tried and failed. The payoff for being a hero is high, but, when other qualified people could not handle the job—new managers must be careful not to slip on their egos. A clearer and proven path is more sensible and less fraught with uncertainties and danger. Here, again, objectives come into play, however, since some people find the proven ladders less appealing than the greased flag pole.

CASE STUDY

Trouble at Triangle

Dr. John Porter is one of 20 full-time physicians employed at Triangle Hospital, a 600-bed university teaching hospital in Metroplex. Porter's specialty is gastroenterology, and he is generally regarded as a competent physician. Indeed in the 14 years that he has been at Triangle, not a single complaint has ever been lodged against him. He is clearly one of the informal social leaders of the medical staff. For example, he plays viola in a chamber music group that he founded nine years ago, and he has numerous friends on the medical staff. Also, he has been happy to use his political connections (his father was once mayor of Metroplex) to benefit the hospital and its staff. Three years ago, Porter went through a traumatic divorce, in which he lost a bitter custody fight over his children.

Last year, a housekeeper making a routine Sunday evening check of the physicians' offices found Porter's office in disarray. She straightened it up and on Monday reported this unusual situation to the executive housekeeper. The following Sunday evening, the office was again in disarray, but this time a needle and syringe were found in the wastepaper basket. The housekeeper reported her findings to the executive housekeeper, who brought the situation to the attention of the assistant director and director of Triangle. After a few minutes of discussion, the executive housekeeper was told to have the housekeeper retrieve the needle and syringe if it happened again. Also, the hospital director asked for the emergency room roster for the past two weekends and asked the Medical Records Department for a run-down on Porter's cases for the past two weeks. Both sources indicated that he had not seen patients over the weekend. On a hunch that Porter may have seen a private patient during that period, he checked with Porter's business office—but that turned up nothing.

During the next week, the director casually asked Porter's colleagues about his general state of health—physical and mental. Responses from the staff indicated no problems. The following Monday, another report was delivered about a "messed up office," but this time the syringe and needle were retrieved. The director sent them to the laboratory for examination, where they were found to have been used with morphine. The director then briefed the hospital's chief of medical staff on the entire situation. The chief said he would talk to Porter. The following is the transcript of the conversation:

Chief: John, how are you feeling?
Porter: Fine, why do you ask?
Chief: Well, you look tired lately, maybe even a bit depressed.
Porter: Yes, I'm tired, but that's because I've been working my butt off.
Chief: Are you depressed?
Porter: No, why? What are you getting at?
Chief: O.K. I won't beat around the bush. The housekeepers found morphine in your office during the weekend and your office has been messed up. What's going on?
Porter: Oh, well, my pet golden retriever, you know, Lassie, has terminal cancer, so I've been giving her morphine to ease the pain.
Chief: Is that all?
Porter: Yes.

The chief went back to the director with Porter's story, adding that, in his opinion, Porter was not telling the truth. The director and chief decided to put Porter under close surveillance for the next few weeks in order to see how he was dealing with his patients. No major problems were observed, although reports from the nursing staff indicated that he was more short-tempered than usual and the business office indicated that his patient load seemed to be slowly decreasing. His appearance was generally neat, although he did come to the hospital on a few occasions without a shave and in badly wrinkled clothes. Only once during this four-week period was a syringe and needle found in his office. During this time, however, the housekeeper reported that Porter has personally installed another lock on the inside of the door.

The chief and director again met and decided that Porter represented too great a threat and that he needed a sabbatical to straighten out his problem. The director called Porter in.

Director:	John, how are you feeling?
Porter:	Fine, but why the hell all this interest in my health here?
Director:	John, I'm concerned about you. Are you into drugs?
Porter:	No!
Director:	So why the needles and syringes with morphine? Look, we want to help you.
Porter:	I told the chief my dog is dying of cancer, and you can help by just leaving me alone.
Director:	Look, John, I think you need a rest.
Chief:	I agree with the director. We want you to take a two-month sabbatical with pay and get yourself together.
Porter:	I am together.
Director:	We don't want a big hassle here. If you want to stay at Triangle, we want you to take a sabbatical and see a psychiatrist during that time.
Porter:	Do I have a choice?
Chief:	Not really.
Porter:	O.K.—I'll go.

After Porter left, the director and chief reviewed the situation. They both felt that Porter was into drugs, and their solution was reasonable.

Two months later, the director received Porter's letter of resignation from the medical staff.

A year later, a letter came from a hospital in another state asking for a recommendation from the hospital director and chief of the medical staff for "Dr. John Porter, whom we wish to appoint as Chief of Gastroenterology at our hospital."

Discussion Questions

1. What alternatives could the chief and director have pursued? What are the implications of these alternatives?
2. What should be the response of the chief of staff and the hospital director to the request for a recommendation?

NOTES

1. W.B. Cornell, *Organization and Management in Industry and Business* (New York: Ronald Press, 1947), p. 46.
2. J.L. Gibson, J.M. Ivancevich, and J.H. Donnelly, *Organizations* (Dallas, TX: Business Pub. Inc., 1979), p. 40.
3. P. Drucker, *Management* (New York: Harper & Row, 1973), p. XIII.
4. Ibid., pp. 419-429.
5. *Fortune,* "In the News," February 12, 1979, p. 16.
6. *Fortune,* "Candid Reflections of a Businessman in Washington," January 29, 1979, pp. 36-49.
7. W.D. Guth, and R. Tagiuri, "Personal Values and Corporate Strategies," *Harvard Business Review* 43, no. 3 (September-October:123-132.
8. J. Hahn, "Ethical Conduct of the CEO," *Hospital Progress* 56, No. 11 (November):36-40.
9. Drucker, *Management,* pp. 405-410.

Chapter 6

The Board of Directors

Boards of directors are a fact of life for managers of corporations—health care and otherwise. State statutes usually set some requirements for corporate boards, such as age or number of members on the board. These same statutes then enfranchise the board with the legal responsibility and authority for the operation of the enterprise. The board, in turn, normally delegates significant amounts of their powers to a full-time managerial staff headed by a chief executive officer.

BOARD FUNCTIONS

In discussing the board's function, Heen identifies eight areas for Board activity:

(a) policy decisions with respect to products, services, prices, wages, labor relations; (b) selection, supervision and removal of officers and possibly other management personnel; (c) fixing of executive compensations, pension/retirement, etc. plans: (d) determination of dividends, financing and capital changes; (e) delegation of authority for administrative and possibly other action; (f) possible adoption, amendment and repeal of by-laws; (g) possible participation, along with shareholders, in approving various extraordinary corporate matters; and (h) supervision and vigilance for the welfare of the whole enterprise.[1]

While some of these functions are irrelevant for not-for-profit health care organizations, most of the responsibilities are appropriate for the health care organization board member.

The problem of board effectiveness and involvement is common to all organizations. For example, when the famous bankruptcies of W.T. Grant, Lockheed, and

Penn Central Railroad occurred, who claimed to be uninformed? The board! Does it seem possible that board members of major industrial concerns, the elite of America's business establishment, could be so unaware?

Drucker, in his book *Management,* titles a chapter "Needed: An Effective Board." He argues that boards by their very nature, ambiguity of mission, and divergence of interest, are preprogrammed for failure.[2] A common experience in health care is that of finding executives whose performance is excellent in business but who cannot function effectively on the board of a not-for-profit organization. This can be understood, in part, if the composition of boards—health care or industrial—is considered. Data from a Heidrick and Struggles study of directors indicate that most board members are well into middle age (the average age being 57), that most people are selected for their personal or professional stature, that a person's functional area of expertise is a second but significantly less important reason for selection, and that availability is a considerably less important reason in selection.[3]

In a study of 134 boards of Health Systems Agencies (HSAs)—organizations that operate under strict federal guidelines calling for a membership that is "broadly representative" of the communities being served—it was found that:

> *65 percent of the board members were classified in professional and managerial positions,* 10 percent in the remaining occupational categories (e.g., clerical), and 22 percent were not in the civilian labor force (persons formerly employed who were housewives, disabled, and so on). For executive committees, the figures for these categories were 75 percent, 7 percent and 17 percent respectively. In contrast, 1970 Census data indicated that 13 percent of the experienced civilian labor force were in professional and managerial occupations, 45 percent in the remaining occupational categories and 42 percent were classified as not in the civilian labor force. Thus, the higher-status occupational groups were extremely overrepresented while persons of lower-status occupational groups and not in the civilian labor force were extremely underrepresented. This underrepresentation was even greater for the executive committees.[4]

This is a pattern seen almost universally in the health care field. A review of a typical Board membership (with the exclusion of community-based programs such as a neighborhood health center) is like reading the who's who of an area. Boards generally are not representative of any group other than the upper middle class of the community. The justification for this skewed representation is that such a group is likely to bring greater financial and intellectual resources to a board. Addressing this issue of board composition in an amusing article, Chandler suggests (somewhat backhandedly) that a balanced board must be the goal, with various criteria being evaluated "from the subjective—candor, enthusiasm, manner of presentation (articulation and appearance), willingness to serve community, cooperativeness; to the more objective—age, occupation, standing in the community, place of residence, etc.''[5]

BOARD MANAGEMENT RELATIONS

For the manager, the fundamental question is; How can a manager have an effective relationship with a board? At one extreme, the manager must cope with a necessary evil; at another, the manager is able to utilize the resources that a board can offer. Many managers view their relationship with their board as something of an adversary one. This was well articulated by J. Peter Grace, the chief executive of the multi-billion dollar W.R. Grace conglomerate, when he said, "Do you mean to tell me that if I work 100 hours a week for 4.3 weeks a month on average so that I'm working 430 hours a month, some guy is going to come in and in three or four hours outsmart me? I mean that's crazy! No matter how smart you are, if I work 100 times harder than you on a given subject you have no way of catching me.''[6] As a reflection of this perspective, Grace's boardroom does not have the traditional conference table but rather is arranged more like a college classroom. In dealing with his board, Grace states that he keeps them fully informed; for example, for one month's meeting he provided them with a report that was over 400 pages long.

Is this typical? In the Heidrick and Struggles study, it appeared that most companies provided their directors with only minutes of previous meetings, some financial data, and an agenda before board meetings. In most cases, no summaries of board committee meetings subsequent to the last board meetings, marketing data, or data to support agenda items were provided. It can be concluded that only those board members who are involved with committees, which is usually the group making critical decisions, or those who are extremely well informed about agenda items can offer much of worth at a given meeting. In the Grace example, it must be recognized that without an independent staff or a major investment of their own time, board members would find it impossible to digest or evaluate critically the 400 pages sent out to the Board. Management then, through its control of information to the board de facto, has a major impact on the effectiveness and value of the board.

In health care organizations, it appears that effective relationships are of major concern. For example, in a 1980 review article on governance, Umbdenstock notes that

> for hospital trustees, administrators and physicians, many of the same issues in hospital governance remained in the forefront throughout the '70s. What are the board's proper roles and responsibilities? What are

the proper relationships with management and the medical staff? What about the board's need to represent the community? Who ultimately directs the institution and how do trustees ensure the quality of care provided in the hospital?[7]

The U.S. Chamber of Commerce, in its 1974 publication *A Primer for Hospital Trustees,* cautions the trustees about their balance of involvement—that is, how can they set policy and stay out of implementation?[8] The administrative perspective and concerns are perhaps best identified in a 1973 document from the American College of Hospital Administrators titled *Principles of Appointment and Tenure of Executive Officers.* In it, the authors noted that "some board members in some hospitals cross over into line management, consciously or unconsciously."[9] When that in fact occurs, directors represent potential adversaries. As a preventive medicine measure then, the behavior suggested by Grace is almost a necessity for survival.

In a 1974 study sponsored by the Macy Foundation, *The Governance of Voluntary Teaching Hospitals in New York City,* Nelson, the former president of Johns Hopkins Hospital, found the major teaching hospitals in New York City facing many serious problems, some of which related to the board:

- Confusion of authority in governance, management and medical staffs resulting from the duality of mission of the teaching hospital, which faces toward the medical school in the performance of its teaching and learning functions, and toward the community and its doctors' patients in the performance of its service functions.

- Boards of trustees which are predominantly white, male, and business-oriented, with only token representation of other interests.

- Board leadership concentrated in small, entrenched groups complacent about the quality of their leadership.

- Except for leadership groups, board membership poorly informed about hospital goals and problems and uninformed about outside forces impinging on hospitals.

- Trustees frustrated by lack of information and involvement but nervous about getting involved in financial and medical problems.

- Chief executives who lack the authority and backing required for effective negotiation with outside forces and effective control of medical affairs.

- Administrative staffs which are generally strong at top level but lack depth of expertise in finance, law, medical staff organization and other specialties.

- Communities mistrustful of institutional goals and critical of institutional services.

- Lack of any standards of performance for hospital trustees or methods of evaluating quality and effectiveness of governance.[10]

The picture of boards painted by Nelson and the others is gloomy indeed. Who or what is responsible for this state of events? Some easy answers might be that boards are picked for the wrong reasons—a person who has the prestige but lacks the time might be selected over someone with the time but limited prestige. Potential economic resource people (i.e., Mr. Gotrocks, who might leave money for a building) may be more important than those with expertise and interest. Some managers may want weak boards—and uninformed boards are weak.

On the other hand, strong boards can play dramatic leadership roles for organizations. Individually and collectively, they can represent and promote the organization's interest; they can serve as a sounding board or as a review and comment mechanism for innovation; and, finally, with proper development, they can serve as the major organizational evaluation mechanism.

KNOWLEDGE AND UNDERSTANDING OF DIRECTORS

Several years ago, a group of 26 senior health administrators were asked what they thought were the most important things directors could know or understand about the health system and about the role of the manager. Responses to the question concerning knowledge and understanding of the health system varied widely. Some managers wanted their boards to be focused on national affairs, looking at the broad legislative and policy issues, and planning alternative health systems; others were more interested in having directors focused on the role their own organization might play in a community or in developing quality services. A conceptual construct could be that some managers view the board as an external reporting and sounding panel, while others see it as part of the internal drive mechanism of the organization.

When this same group of managers considered what they wanted the directors to know and understand about the manager's job, there was considerably less variance. Virtually all of the managers wanted their directors to know and understand more about the problems of managing professionals (most notably physicians) and the fiscal problems of their respective organizations. Additionally, a number of managers felt it was important that board members understand the importance of delegating authority and responsibility—a particularly troubling notion, considering that many board members do not delegate authority in their own organizations.

BEHAVIOR OF DIRECTORS

Several types of behavior can be considered desirable in a director. A board member must be active and participate in the board meetings, as well as in the committee structure. The director who shows up occasionally and must always be "updated" wastes everyone's time and can be counterproductive. The director who wants to learn more and seeks additional expertise is respected by other directors and management. This interest should be construed as an indication that the director supports the organization, and such a person should be considered a major asset. Seeking additional responsibility is another important behavior, since it is a sign of commitment. An individual who follows through is invaluable. Board members who offer suggestions and ideas but simply do not deliver are not nearly as helpful as those who develop their programs. In general then, the useful and effective director is one who is conscientious, thoughtful, articulate, concerned, and available—a tall order indeed.

Undesirable behaviors could, in many instances, lead to a managerial Armageddon or revolution. At the top of the undesirable list is the demanding board person who involves management with inconsequential work activities or focuses attention on trivial matters. The President of one hospital board had the assistant director trailing after her carrying a sample book of fabrics so that the $25,000 per year manager could hold the samples against various couches throughout the hospital and the President could choose the new fabrics. A morning doing that is demeaning and demoralizing to a manager, as well as a waste of money.

Vying for the top of the list is the board member who has accepted the position for personal gain. This gain comes in various guises. At worst, there are board members who, despite conflict-of-interest laws, want to do business with the organization on whose board they serve. Sometimes being on a board works to their advantage in their own businesses; for example, one restaurateur who served as treasurer on the board of a large hospital insisted that the hospital use certain purveyors—the same ones he used. Subsequently, he received discounts from these purveyors for his own business. A less overt personal gain is seen when a person joins a board for the experience or "service" credits necessary to advance in the home organization.

The directors who may disturb managers most are those who like to end-run management. For example, they might make commitments without consulting management, or they might stir up enthusiasm for a new program without investigating it or discussing it with staff. When a policy is adopted that they object to, however, they respond by openly criticizing management and the board.

Small thinking is a characteristic of many board members. Along with this is a tendency to focus on a "hobbyhorse." For example, a board member whose pet project is the snack bar might insist on an overinvestment by management in a program that should really have a lower priority.

The naive, uninformed, and lazy director is also a problem. Again, such a director expends energy, which is limited, for insignificant issues.

BOARD DEVELOPMENT

Boards are valuable assets for a health care organization—but they must be properly selected and nurtured. The right people must be selected. Here, myth must be distinguished from reality. For every story about a board person who gave a building, there are a hundred other stories about someone whom "we thought would give a building, died, and gave nothing." Organizations should approach the selection of directors with considerable seriousness and select only those people who enhance the value of the organization because of their expertise, availability, and, yes—in some cases, personal stature. Considered in this decision should be the question, If time and effort are invested in this person, will there be a return on that investment? A negative answer suggests that the search process should be continued.

Having selected the right people, the organization must then make an investment. This investment has several dimensions. First, the manager should learn as much as possible about the new director and that director's home organization, experience, or profession. This includes an assessment of areas of strength and weakness. Doing this diagnostic workup demonstrates an interest in the board member's professional and personal development, while simultaneously permitting an evaluation of how and where the new director can fit into the organizational scheme. Second, the board member must be educated in the major issues and problems faced in the health industry, in general, and the particular component, specifically. In doing this, it is not necessary to focus on detail as much as to look at issues and options. Finally, the board member has to keep informed.

The strategy of overwhelming the board, as Grace does, is not likely to result in an interested, involved, and supportive board. On the other hand, a board that is tuned in to an organization can be invaluable for both the organization's and the manager's success.

CASE STUDY

The Tri-County Health Council Case

The Tri-County Health Council became a federally designated HSA 18 months ago. The area covered by the agency has a total population of 637,400 people, 80 percent of whom are located in two metropolitan areas: Calvin City, with 311,000 people, and Fair Harbor, with 209,000 residents. The remaining population is scattered throughout the relatively rural region. Calvin City is an old industrial city, while Fair Harbor developed after World War II as a center for high technology electronic firms. The area has two large teaching hospitals. One is in Fair Harbor at the state university medical school, and the other, Calvin Community Hospital, is in Calvin and is under church auspices.

The Health Council, while theoretically a new organization, had its roots in the former tri-county hospital association; indeed, the present council director is the former Tri-County Comprehensive Health Planning Director. For nine years prior to that, he was the hospital association director.

The present Health Council governing body consists of 60 people, 31 of whom are considered consumers. The remaining members fit the appropriate guideline categories (Exhibit 6-1). An executive committee of 15 members who meet twice each month has also been established according to federal guidelines.

The director believes that the board is ineffective. He is concerned about their lack of preparation for meetings (which are held nine times per year), the amount of irrelevant discussion at board meetings, the quality of the dialogue at meetings, and finally, the amount of time he and his staff spend between meetings with board members on trivial issues.

Two recent examples involved a computerized axial tomography (CAT) scanner and ambulatory surgery. In the CAT scanner case, the HSA denied certificate-of-need approval to one of the four hospitals in Fair Harbor. The hospital involved was Orange Hospital, a 250-bed non-teaching hospital operated by the same church that has a large teaching hospital in Calvin City. The situation was complicated by the fact that the legislation then in effect required a certificate-of-need only for projects in excess of $150,000; the hospital's CAT scanner cost only $75,000 (it was a used machine purchased from the church's sister hospital in Fair Harbor). Subsequent to the purchase and installation of the CAT scanner, legislation was passed in the state bringing CAT scanner installation under certificate-of-need requirements, regardless of cost—and the legislation was enacted retrospectively.

The net result of this was a major conflict between Orange Hospital and the HSA. Board members were split on this issue; some consumers felt that all the technology should not be centered in teaching hospitals, and others argued that there were already too many CAT scanners in the area and another one would drive up health care costs. Supporters of Calvin also got into the argument on the grounds that "their" hospital should not become a stepchild institution. During this period, the director of the HSA remained "above the controversy" and did not take any public position. Privately, however, he lobbied against approval of the certificate of need. He felt frustrated that the board's consumers were so divided on this issue, and he was disappointed when he was publicly accused of trying to manipulate the board.

Exhibit 6-1 Federal Legislation on Governing Boards: P.L. 93-641, As Amended

Governing Body.

(A) A health systems agency which is a public regional planning body or unit of general local government shall, in addition to any other governing body, have a governing body for health planning, which is established in accordance with subparagraph (C), which shall have the responsibilities prescribed in subparagraph (B), and which has exclusive authority to perform for the agency the functions described in section 300L—2 of this title. Any other health systems agency shall have a governing body composed, in accordance with subparagraph (C), of not less than ten members and of not more than thirty members, except that the number of members may exceed thirty if the governing body has established another unit (referred to in this paragraph as an "executive committee") composed, in accordance with subparagraph (C), of not more than twenty-five members of the governing body and has delegated to that unit the authority to take such action (other than the establishment and revision of the plans referred to in subparagraph (B) (ii)) as the governing body is authorized to take.

(B) The governing body—

(i) shall be responsible for the internal affairs of the health systems agency, including matters relating to the staff of the agency, the agency's budget, and procedures and criteria (developed and published pursuant to section 300n—1 of this title) applicable to its functions under subsections (e), (f), (g), and (h) of section 300L—2 of this title;

(ii) shall be responsible for the establishment of the health systems plan and annual implementation plan required by section 300L—2 (b) of this title;

(iii) shall be responsible for the approval of grants and contracts made and entered into under section 300L—2 (c) (3) of this title;

(iv) shall be responsible for the approval of all actions taken pursuant to subsections (e), (f), (g), and (h), of section 300L—2 of this title;

Exhibit 6-1 continued

    (v) shall (I) issue an annual report concerning the activities of the agency, (II) include in that report the health systems plan and annual implementation plan developed by the agency, and a listing of the agency's income, expenditures, assets, and liabilities, and (III) make the report readily available to the residents of the health service area and the various communications media serving such area;

    (vi) shall meet at least once in each calendar quarter of a year and shall meet at least two additional times in a year unless its executive committee meets at least twice in that year; and

    (vii) shall (I) conduct its business meetings in public, (II) give adequate notice to the public of such meetings, and (III) make its records and data available, upon request, to the public.

The governing body (and executive committee (if any)) of a health systems agency shall act only by vote of a majority of its members present and voting at a meeting called upon adequate notice to all of its members and at which a quorum is in attendance. A quorum for a governing body and executive committee shall be not less than one-half of its members.

    (C) The membership of the governing body and the executive committee (if any) of an agency shall meet the following requirements:

    (i) A majority (but not more than 60 percent of the members) shall be residents of the health service area served by the entity who are consumers of health care and who are not (nor within the twelve months preceding appointment been) providers of health care and who are broadly representative of the social, economic, linguistic and racial populations, geographic areas of the health service area, and major purchasers of health care.

    (ii) The remainder of the members shall be residents of the health service area served by the agency who are providers of health care and who represent (I) physicians (particularly practicing physicians), dentists, nurses, optometrists, and other health professionals, (II) health care institutions (particularly hospitals, long-term care facilities, substance abuse treatment facilities, and health maintenance organizations), (III) health

Exhibit 6-1 continued

care insurers, (IV) health professional schools, and (V) the allied health professions. Not less than one-third of the providers of health care who are members of the governing body or executive committee of a health systems agency shall be direct providers of health care (as described in section 300n (3) of this title).

(iii) The membership shall—

    (I) include (either through consumer or provider members) public elected officials and other representatives of governmental authorities in the agency's health service area and representatives of public and private agencies in the area concerned with health.

    (II) include a percentage of individuals who reside in nonmetropolitan areas within the health service area which percentage is equal to the percentage of residents of the area who reside in nonmetropolitan areas, and

    (III) if the health systems agency serves an area in which there is located one or more hospitals or other health care facilities of the Veterans' Administration, include, as an ex officio member, an individual whom the Chief Medical Director of the Veterans' Administration shall have designated for such purpose, and if the agency serves an area in which there is located one or more qualified health maintenance organizations (within the meaning of section 300e—9 of this title), include at least one member who is representative of such organizations.

(iv) If, in the exercise of its functions, a governing body or executive committee appoints a subcommittee of its members or an advisory group, it shall, to the extent practicable, make its appointments to any such subcommittee or group in such a manner as to provide the representation on such subcommittee or group described in this subparagraph.

In the second case, one of the subarea boards recommended the development of free-standing ambulatory surgery centers in the region. This recommendation was reviewed and approved by the board in principle, and a study committee was set up. After three months of activity, the committee produced a document that the director considered "useless . . . full of rhetoric . . . non specific." He was particularly irked by one recommendation that the centers be used for acupuncture.

The present table of organization at the agency is shown in Figure 6-1. The HSA's total budget for fiscal year 1980 was $400,000. The Director of Public Information has board development as a prime responsibility. To date, this has involved personalized one-day orientation discussions, tours for each of the new members (15-20 per year), and the preparation of a newsletter.

Discussion Questions

1. What topics should be included in an educational program for the board?
2. How can the success (or failure) of such a program be evaluated?
3. What else (other than education) could be causing the Director's problems?

Figure 6-1 Organization of the Tri-County Health Council

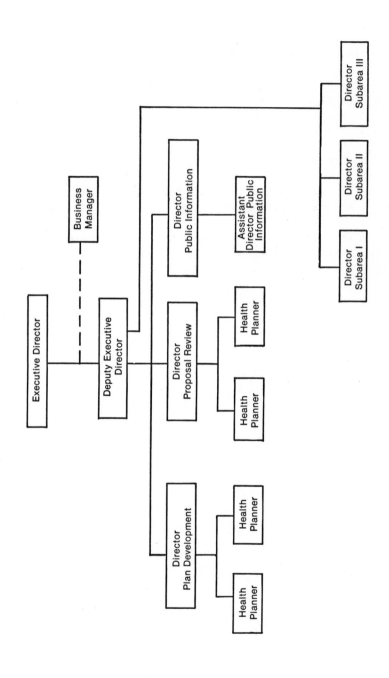

NOTES

1. H.G. Heen, *Handbook of the Law of Corporations* (St. Paul, MN: West Pub. Co., 1970), p. 415.
2. P. Drucker, *Management* (New York: Harper & Row, 1973), pp. 627-636.
3. Heidrick and Struggles, *The Changing Board* (1975), p. 5.
4. U.S. Department of Health, Education and Welfare, *Project Summary, Board and Staff Composition of Health Planning Agencies,* HRA Pub. No. 78-609, 1978, p. 10.
5. R.L. Chandler, "Filling Empty Board Seats," *Hospital and Health Services Administration* 25, no. 1 (Winter 1980):85.
6. "Peter Grace's Love-Hate Relationship With His Board," *Forbes,* May 15, 1976, p. 76.
7. R.J. Umbdenstock, "Governance: A Decade of Steady Growth," *Trustees* 33 (1980):17.
8. U.S. Chamber of Commerce, *A Primer for Hospital Trustees* (Washington, DC:1974), p. 25.
9. American College of Hospital Administrators, *Principles of Appointment and Tenure of Executive Officers* (Chicago, 1973), p. 4.
10. The Macy Foundation, *The Governance of Voluntary Teaching Hospitals in New York City* (New York, 1974), pp. 8-9.

Chapter 7

Motivation

The McCormick Spice Company of Baltimore was one of the pioneers in participative management, the art and science of involving all levels of employees in decision making so that employees become committed to the future of the organization. The company itself credited its survival through the Depression to this type of participation.[1] In 1967, I had the opportunity to tour the Baltimore factory with the late Charles McCormick. After taking me on a walk through the main plant during which he greeted a number of long-time employees by first names and exchanged pleasantries about their families, he said to me in a rather somber tone that it seemed that the work force was changing in a most unsatisfactory way. He felt that, in the past, people were really concerned about job security and being part of a company where top management was concerned about their welfare. Today, he noted, the work force seemed more interested in paychecks and less interested in security. For example, he could not understand why young people were willing to quit jobs after only a few weeks. In his mind, a job was analogous to a career.

So what was happening at McCormick? Why the high turnover? Why the problems in motivation? On one hand, the organization's environment was impressive. This was perhaps best exemplified by the personnel department, which was called the Department of Human Relations, and its motto, displayed in foot-high letters at the intersection of the walls and ceiling: "Know all ye that enter here have faith not fear." Clearly, the executives had a genuine interest and commitment to the theory and practice of participative management. On the other hand, it was clear that there was a generation gap in their work force. The old-time employees were people of the Depression to whom their brand of participative management was important, while the new work force was composed of high-school graduates, most of whom had been born after World War II. In the McCormick case, it appeared that major social events, plus the changing demography and economics of Baltimore—certainly not the good intentions of the

101

company—had been affecting a carefully developed strategy for employee motivation that had been successful for a number of years.

In other for-profit firms such as the department store, the manager is at the top of the organization, and each member of that organization works toward the "bottom line" goals of the store, which are quite clear. Because each person is not an individual entrepreneur, but rather part of a team, effort is toward goal achievement and that achievement is measurable. Large elements of the work force are interchangeable and dispensable, since only limited training and experience are required for the job. Finally, the work force is generally nonprofessional and is responding to organizational rather than professional needs.

The community hospital, in contrast, employs a rather heterogeneous group, ranging from physicians to janitors. Education, social class, and age differences are significant, and job functions vary from those that require a great deal of knowledge and are rather intellectual in nature to those that require practically no knowledge but are physically demanding. This complex situation is further complicated by the continual interaction and interdependence of these people and the somewhat unclear bottom line of a hospital's activities. Finally, the key personnel, community physicians, are independent contractors who utilize the facility and its resources to enrich themselves intellectually and economically but do not reimburse the institution for its support of their activities; rather, the costs are simply transferred directly to the consumer, in this case, the patient.

The complexity of the hospital situation is well illustrated in the operating room. The procedure is performed by a surgeon, probably a white male who is a private practitioner and is billing the patient privately for the procedure. The operating room clothes he wears, the instruments he uses, the facility and other supplies utilized all belong to the hospital. An anesthesiologist, who is also billing the patient privately, is likewise a private entrepreneur who utilizes hospital-owned equipment, which is likely to have been purchased at his request. The scrub nurse, the circulating nurses, and the other supportive personnel in the operating room are hospital employees. The nurses are likely to be women graduates of a two-, three-, or four-year nursing program with some on-the-job training for their specialized duties in the operating room. The physicians are all college graduates, medical school graduates, and have completed extensive three-, four- or five-year surgical training postgraduate programs. If a specimen such as a frozen section has to be analyzed during the procedure or an x-ray taken and read, another group of people are needed: the technicians in the laboratory or x-ray department, plus the pathologists and radiologists. This last group of physicians may have a complex financial arrangement with the institution in which their salaries are related to a percentage of the revenues generated by their respective departments. Again, the facility provides the lion's share of the resources necessary for the department to generate its revenues.

Between cases, the operating room is scrubbed clean by a group of housekeeping employees. These are likely to be high-school graduates with minimal training; in most cases, they are from a considerably lower socioeconomic class than the physicians and nurses. Scheduling for operating room time is handled by either a hospital-employed clerk or nurse under the general direction of the administration.

What motivates the operating room crew? Is the surgeon motivated in the same way as the anesthesiologist, the nurse, the operating room supervisor, and the housekeeping employee?

The central dilemma in terms of motivation is that a heterogeneous group is likely to have different needs and aspirations. The managerial goal must be to set a tone in the managerial environment whereby people can simultaneously meet their personal aspirations and satisfy organizational objectives.

This goal is extremely difficult to attain for two major reasons. First, organizations are fundamentally impersonal; jobs in organizations are designed to fit the organization's needs and then tailored to fit the particular people. It is somewhat analogous to renting formal wear. The sleeves are raised a bit and the trousers shortened; the next week the trousers are lengthened and the waist taken in a bit. Rarely do large organizations go out of business because someone leaves or dies. Second, from the organization's perspective, jobs have to be designed, structured, and assigned. Work has to be done on a structured basis and in an orderly manner. The housekeeping employees cannot scrub down the operating room when it fits into their schedule, and the food service employees cannot deliver the meals at their convenience. Thus, somewhere within the hospital organization, priorities must be set, and these priorities dictate the resources, human and nonhuman, necessary to meet these goals.

Conflict is inherent in the process of simultaneously meeting both personal and organizational goals, since personal needs are inevitably made subordinate to major organizational goals. For example, the hospital must function 24 hours per day. Who shall staff the institution on the least desirable shifts? Although the organization can provide extra financial compensation for working on Thanksgiving or Christmas, is the money a substitute for time?

ATTITUDE AND BEHAVIOR

Attitude and behavior are not synonymous terms, and a person's attitude toward something or even beliefs are not necessarily reliable predictors of that person's behavior. An attitude refers to a person's feelings, perhaps interests, not to an overt act, which is behavior. Much research lately has been done in the area of factors that have an impact on work satisfaction. The importance of this research lies in the assumption that a more satisfied worker is likely to be a "better" worker, which usually means a more efficient and effective worker.

Such an association between satisfaction and performance has not always been observed in the research on the relationship between attitude and behavior. A classic example is the 1934 work of LaPierre, who undertook an inquiry about the attitude and behavior of Americans toward Japanese; he demonstrated the lack of congruence between attitude and behavior.[2] Subsequent research suggests that attitude may be only one of many intervening variables that are related to behavior and that the association is not necessarily direct.[3] Managers must carefully examine not only the attitudes but also the behavior of their staff. In the process, they must examine their own attitudes and behavior concerning their job, their staff, and the goals to be achieved, since all of these factors are likely to have an impact on the managerial processes used to reach goals as well as the final outcomes.

HIERARCHY OF NEEDS

One of the most important conceptual contributions to our understanding of motivation was made by Maslow when he presented his theory on the hierarchy of needs. He assumed that people's needs are hierarchical in nature and are met on a step-wise basis. Thus, the lowest level need must be met before an individual can move on to the need at the next step, and so forth. While his assumptions have been frequently commented upon and criticized, the basic categorization of needs has widely been acknowledged and often accepted.[4,5]

Maslow postulated that the lowest level of need was physiological: the need for bread and water. When a person is deprived of the means to meet this need, nothing else appears to be important. This need is not usually a concern of managers, since the general attitude is that most people have "enough" to fulfill their basic physiological needs. These needs have a tendency to shift as expectations grow higher, however. One person's castle is another's shack; an acceptable standard of living for one person is too low for another. A former government health official said in *The New York Times* that an important reason for his resignation from a $45,000 per year job was that he could not afford to live on that salary. Two children in an expensive private college and one in private school made a $45,000 salary insufficient for that person. Most people would find such a salary a considerable improvement, but the person in question felt that his basic needs were not being met.

Maslow's second level need is that for security and safety. Managers have commonly perceived this to mean that people need to know that no physical or psychological harm will result from their work. This concept has within it the notion of equity or fairness; if workers feel that they are being treated fairly, their needs are being met. In this author's interpretation, it also refers to a person's feeling of insulation against the stress of transitions. In the health field, this is particularly significant because of the widespread use of government monies to fund delivery programs. Those working in the health industry at almost any level need to know the probable impact of growth, development, or winding down on their future. Unfortunately, those individuals with the least mobility are likely to be the ones who feel the greatest impact of any program change.

The third level has been defined as social, sometimes "love." An individual has a need to belong to and identify with a group and an organization. The recruiting techniques of the Marine Corps in the 1970s were based on this need. With the assistance of the J. Walter Thompson marketing firm, they advertised for "A Few Good Men." Belong to a select group—belong! An interesting example of this in the health field involved a hospital in Brooklyn, New York. At the suggestion of the chairman of the Board of Trustees, all hospital staff were required to wear white coats. Despite the expense of clothing hundreds of employees and the burden on the laundry of keeping the coats clean, it gave the staff an unusual sense of belonging as well as professionalism, at least superficially.

The fourth level on Maslow's hierarchy is that of esteem. People must be recognized by their peers and supervisors as important contributors to the organization. They also need self-recognition, a rather complicated issue, since numerous perfectly competent people lack confidence (and occasionally, quite confident people lack competence—a different sort of problem). Some people in organizations simply cannot recognize their self-worth, despite external acknowledgment. Because of their rigid educational barriers to "advancement" in health care organizations, there are often problems with satisfying an individual's need for esteem. For example, state and federal laws prevent the upgrading of the world's best nursing aide to a licensed practical nurse or registered nurse. The world's finest nurse-midwife is stymied in advancement without a medical degree.

The highest level of need, Maslow suggests, is that of "self-actualization." In today's parlance this means that a person is truly "turned on" by what they do. In a sense, they have become a totally integrated person; they have interlaced their personal and work lives and are thoroughly "enjoying" both. Examples most often used when talking of self-actualized persons are dead artists and musicians such as Beethoven or Van Gogh. Rarely has anyone suggested that a bolt tightener on the Ford assembly line at the River Rouge plant was self-actualized, nor the foreman or even the supervisor. Perhaps the plant manager was self-actualized, and certainly Henry Ford II was!

As noted earlier, an underlying assumption of Maslow's was that self-actualization is impossible before these other hurdles are cleared. Consider again the example of the health official who earned $45,000 per year. He loved his job, despite his personal need for security and the job's inherent insecurity, since it was a political appointment; he received tremendous ego satisfaction from the job, but it did not satisfy more basic needs—thus the resignation. This example suggests that the levels are useful handles when various discreet reasons for motivation are considered, but they may not interact as postulated in this theory.

Finally, certain of these needs appear to be more critical than others; for example, many people work in non-ego-satisfying jobs for the security that they offer. In addition, certain of Maslow's defined needs require satisfaction only at a minimal level. Occasionally, however, specific needs predominate; for example, in times of personal stress an individual may find it most important to be in a low risk, high security type job. At other times, the high risk, potentially high payoff job may be more appealing.

Needs are not static. As a person ages, needs shift, become more intense, or change completely. Often, after having attained security, a person no longer values security. Many professional colleagues have resigned once they were granted tenure. The competition and challenge turned them on, not the prize.

MOTIVATION-HYGIENE THEORY

The second major theory of motivation is Herzberg's motivation-hygiene theory.[6] Herzberg suggests that certain job factors serve a motivating function by providing job satisfaction. He notes that "motivation factors that are intrinsic to the job are: achievement, recognition for achievement, the work itself, responsibility and growth and advancement." On the other hand, Herzberg suggests that job dissatisfaction "or hygiene factors that are extrinsic to the job include: company policy and administration, supervision, interpersonal relationships, working conditions, salary, status and security."

According to Herzberg's theory, when people are not dissatisfied, they are not necessarily satisfied; they may be simply not dissatisfied. For example, salary is listed as a hygiene factor. Salary does not really motivate a person but simply prevents that person from being dissatisfied by its level. On the other hand, a sense of being an integral and highly valued person in an organization may produce a highly motivated person.

THEORY X AND THEORY Y

A different and perhaps the most popular concept of motivation was provided by McGregor when he offered his Theory X and Theory Y.[7] Theory X is based on the notion that workers are lazy, indolent, undisciplined or, in today's language, "rip-off artists." To get such people to achieve, a manager must use a reward and punishment approach. For the Theory X manager, a carrot and stick are the two major management tools. Theory Y assumes a different type of worker, one who is mature, responsible, and genuinely interested in doing a fair day's work for a fair day's pay. In this instance, the manager sets a tone and direction for the environment within which the worker achieves.

On the face of it, X appears repugnant, while Y is quite attractive. Indeed, the issue resembles the open classroom/closed classroom debates—one is highly structured, rigid, lacking flexibility and enrichment; the other is open, creative, flexible, and enriched. The problem in all of this is clarity of expectations. Theory Y appears to put a great deal of trust in the worker's ability to set goals and achieve those goals without direction from management. Is this possible? Perhaps it is possible in a highly achieving organization populated by mature, experienced, self-actuated people. However, Drucker points out the disaster that occurred at one major university when a Theory Y-oriented official attempted to use Theory Y management as a vehicle for a revolution in quality at the university. It did not work![8]

Some structure is necessary, and it is useful to the manager and the workers if the goals are clear. This is not to suggest that goals, the inputs needed to achieve those goals, or even the processes of combining those inputs are not negotiable or open to review. But an organization or component without direction is simply confusing itself, everyone around it, and complicating the motivational task of the manager as well as an individual's self-motivational task.

Over the past two decades a number of scholars have advanced other theories of motivation based on observation and research. Many of the newer approaches take a view that motivation is contingent on a number of interacting factors. Some are within the control of managers, but others are clearly outside their purview.

Circumstances do play an important part in a person's need for motivational stimuli and the power of various stimuli. In one organization that I studied a young man who was a department manager "loved" his job. Each morning he reported bright and eager for the day's events, which were heavily developmental in nature. He enjoyed putting the management systems into place and watching them function as he expected. He thrived on contributing to the senior level policy meetings in which decisions that affected his department were made. He tackled staff recruiting with a passion. In his third year, he was bored. He could barely drag himself into the office, and the most petty problem irritated him. He became overbearing with the staff and started shifting his management practices from Theory Y to Theory X. What was going on? Seemingly, everything was functioning in the way he wanted it to function. The systems he developed worked, and the staff he recruited were excellent. When the organization was stable, however, he no longer was challenged. The tumult of a developing organization excited and motivated him; an ongoing operation represented little personal challenge.

Thus, while our limits of understanding motivation can be viewed as an exoneration of anything a manager does, it should be emphasized that understanding human behavior, while a complex task, is indeed the keystone of management. In the previous example, the organization's director called me in order to find candidates for a different innovative senior level post. The idea of recruiting the young man who had already demonstrated his skills had not been considered—he was seemingly content, since he was not complaining.

In the health care field, the task of motivation is exacerbated both because of the nature of the economic relationship between those using the system and the system itself (physicians, patients, and hospitals) and because of the heterogeneity of the work force that must be managed. Typically, health care managers are dealing with professionals, semiprofessionals, and nonprofessionals, and they do not have line or direct authority over all of these people. How does a manager motivate a prima donna surgeon whose behavior is continually fouling up the operating room schedule but whose patient load is an important asset to the institution and who has a strong relationship with the trustees (the manager's boss)? How does a manager get a private practice anesthesiologist on the institution's staff to accept the responsibility for obstetrical anesthesia?

There are no clear-cut solutions to these questions, but they do point out that those in health administration are in the business of motivating key people over whom they have little economic or social control. The two groups affected most are physicians and nurses. A third general group might include the other emerging professionals in the health care organization. To deal more effectively with these groups, it is necessary to understand more about professionalism and the socialization process that these groups undergo.

PROFESSIONALS

In 1933, Carr-Saunders and Wilson identified the three major characteristics of a profession as

1. a lengthy and specialized training that results in the rendering of specialized services to a community
2. an approach to using the specialized techniques that emphasizes the competence and honor of the individuals using the techniques
3. a mechanism for quality control within the profession[9]

In court decisions a definition of profession has been enunciated that defines a profession by the following four parameters:[10]

1. prolonged training
2. work that is predominantly intellectual and varied in character

3. work that requires the exercise of individual discretion
4. work that cannot be standardized in relation to a given period of time

In looking at the physician, Bloom notes that "at the core remains the two primary characteristics: (a) a prolonged specialized training in a body of abstract knowledge, and (b) a service orientation.[11] So American medicine can be defined as a high status occupation that is supposed to be directed toward a social good, theoretically learned, privy to special knowledge and skills, adhering to high ethical standards, and antonomous.

High status is perhaps a result of the other elements. People who have specialized and important knowledge, as well as skills valued by society, are often "awarded" high status. This status in turn attracts other people to make the "sacrifices" necessary to obtain the knowledge and skill necessary to become a professional.

The three traditional professional areas of medicine, law, and the clergy all have a common element; they meet a society need for specialized intermediaries. The medical profession acts as an intermediary between man and the environment and, to an extent, between man and himself. The legal profession functions as the intermediary between man and man or man and society. Finally, the clergy functions as the intermediary between man and the supernatural. It appears that new professions are legitimized at the point where society needs people to interface with some component of society that cannot be handled routinely by the average person. The concept involves control—when man loses or feels unable to establish control over important elements in society, special status and privileges are granted to those individuals who will act for the societal good as controllers of the elements in question.

This concept of controllers can be recognized in the fact that professionals must expend considerable time and effort to acquire the knowledge and skills to practice their professions. Clearly, if the knowledge and skill of any profession could be acquired easily, there would be no reason whatsoever for singling out for special status members of the profession.

Because of their special knowledge and skills, professionals have a contract with society. In the case of medicine, society says "You practice your skills to the best of your ability, and we will give you special privileges." These privileges range from parking a car anywhere to probing the innermost parts of the human body, cutting it up with knives, and injecting a variety of substances into it. Each privilege of a profession is specific. Thus, what is appropriate in the interactions between a lawyer and client differs from what is appropriate between a physician and patient. A final clause of this contract is that society admits that it cannot properly evaluate the quality of the profession's work and therefore the profession itself must take on the major responsibility for evaluating its own functioning. In essence, a profession in the United States effectively controls itself.

Control

The central and one of the most important channels through which the profession exercises its control is undergraduate medical education. Such authors as Hyde and the staff of the *Yale Law Journal* noted that the American Medical Association's Council on Medical Education in fact controls the nation's medical schools; for many years, it has been the actual authority for the licensing of medical schools, although the nominal power rests with the state."[12] The result, Kessel contends, is a natural or franchised monopoly that allows American medicine to regulate their own production.[13]

The second channel of control for the profession is postgraduate medical education. In many states, a one-year internship must be taken after graduation from medical school before new physicians are eligible for licensure. Beyond internships, physicians often desire additional training. Although this training is usually taken with a hospital, it is still subject to approval by one of the review committees of the Council on Medical Education. Licensure, professional status, and privileges rest on an approved internship or residency.

Licensure, the legal sanction to practice provided a physician by the state through its medical practice act, denotes general and sometimes specific qualifications. Prior to the medical licensure acts, individual medical schools or preceptors gave new physicians their "license" to practice medicine. Present licensure, although a state function, is in fact controlled by the medical profession through the state board of medical examiners, the agency that tests and licenses physicians. These boards are composed primarily of physicians, who most often are recommended for their positions by organized medical associations.

Professional status and subsequent privileges, such as entree into the hospital, the main arena of practice, are firmly predicated upon an approved education and postgraduate training. A physician, however, must be trained by profession-approved institutions, in profession-prescribed programs, and must pass profession-designed, profession-administered, and profession-graded examinations. Ultimately, the board of trustees of a hospital grants a physician privileges, but not until the medical board sanctions the appointment. In essence, the board acts as a rubber stamp for the medical staff in these decisions.

In summary then, the medical profession controls itself from the beginning (medical education) to the end (privileges). It is a natural monopoly, although the profession's hold might be loosened if there were appropriate alternatives for physicians.

Some would argue that chiropractors, osteopaths, or even midwives compete with physicians in the health care field. It is well recognized, however, that competitors do not account for a great percentage of the medical care delivered.

Further, such competitors are generally kept outside the medical care system by the medical profession through its privileged societal position as gatekeeper to the system. Physicians sit on the boards of examiners of competing professions, which sometimes include little or no representation from the profession being licensed. Additionally, through their involvement in Blue Cross, Blue Shield, and government reimbursement programs, physicians have made it difficult, if not impossible, to obtain third party payment for services received from competing professions, preventing a large pool of potential patients from using alternative services.

Perhaps most importantly, the physicians are in the dominant position in the utilization of the health facilities of a community. Not only do they control the entrance of their peers into the institutions, but also the entrance of others. For example, nonprofessional midwives or chiropractors can seldom avail themselves of hospital equipment or technology. Essentially, a facility owned by and operated for the community is controlled by a small group to the exclusion of any possible competition.

Central to management's concerns about motivation of the physician is an understanding of their professional value system, which in a major way, it can be argued, determines their likely behavior. What was learned during those early years of training very much shapes the motivation and attitudes toward their own practice and the activities of other health providers that they must interact with in the health system. The basic theoretical framework for this was set out by Parsons.

He suggests that the physician's role can be explained in terms of four pattern variables, i.e., choices that relate to specific motivational and value orientations.[14] The role of physicians, Parsons suggests, is functionally specific; their work relates only to medicine, and technical competence is the keystone of status. In effect, he says that physicians should be and should always strive to remain technically competent. A second attribute is that of neutrality, meaning that the physician should behave in an objective, evaluative, and, in a sense, unemotional manner. The third variable is identified by Parsons as collective orientation. He notes that "the ideology of the profession lays great emphasis on the obligation of the physician to put the welfare of the patient above his personal interest." The final attribute is universalism; physicians must abide by the overall rules of the profession as approved in the specific relationships between them and their patients. In discussing this, Bloom uses the example of euthanasia, "the professional rule about it is the MD's guidepost to his behavior in treating painful terminal illness."

It can be seen that the motivation of professionals requires skills in negotiation and politics, not simply directing. For example, appeals to generalized notions of quality, technical competence, professional standards, and the general well-being of a class of patients are likely to produce more action than economic or political threats (overt or masked).

SEMIPROFESSIONALS AND EMERGING PROFESSIONALS

Large numbers of people working in health organizations could be classified as semiprofessionals or emerging professionals. In many respects, what they do has some of the flavor of a profession: the work is cerebral in nature, the training takes several years after high school, and, in many respects, it is difficult for someone not in the particular field to judge the quality of a person's output. The way our system has been structured, however, these people are not autonomous and must function as part of an organization.

An interesting example of this is the nurse-midwife, a person who has had college and nursing training, postbaccalaureate education, specialized training of from one to two years, and probably considerable experience. In many countries, including most of Western Europe, she (in most cases, the nurse-midwife is a woman) functions as independently as a physician. In the United States, however, she must function under the supervision of a physician and in all but a few instances as part of a larger organization, such as a hospital or clinic, where her role is in large measure defined by the organization.

A cynic could make a convincing argument that the health system teases people with the notion of professionalism. In fact, it may be a way of keeping people in line when, because of the tight structure of the system, there is no way for an individual to advance. Physician's assistants are a case in point.

The professional and emerging professional groups are composed of individuals who, for the most part, have trained in and around the health system and whose jobs, for the most part, are restricted to the health system. For example, the jobs outside of the health system for a nurse, physician, or x-ray technician are quite limited. Others who work in the health system, such as an accountant or house-keeper, could just as easily be working in other parts of the public or private sector. Since their interest and commitment to the health system may be somewhat different from those whose careers are dependent on the system, what interests or motivates them may also be different.

MANAGERIAL APPROACHES TO MOTIVATION

There are several specific managerial approaches to motivation. Fear is perhaps the most widely used (or at least considered) approach. Joseph Heller's statement in his book *Something Happened* should become a classic:

In the office in which I work there are five people of whom I am afraid.
Each of these five people is afraid of four people (excluding overlaps),

for a total of twenty, and each of these twenty people is afraid of six people, making a total of one hundred and twenty people who are feared by at least one person. Each of these one hundred and twenty people is afraid of another one hundred and nineteen, and all of these one hundred and forty-five people are afraid of the twelve men at the top who helped found and build the company and now own and direct it.[15]

Fear is perhaps a derivative of the child-adult conflict many people feel. The boss is the adult; the worker, the child. Workers look to the person in authority for recognition and advancement and, to a large measure, find themselves being defined by the job they have, the organization they work for, and the evaluation they receive from the superior. An interesting and all too prevalent conflicting (and conflicted) managerial type is what the Einstein Associates, an executive recruiting firm, labeled the counterfeit executive: a person who kicks the people below while simultaneously caressing the people above.

Fear certainly works in certain situations, but as a long-run strategy, it is likely to attract and hold the wrong people in an organization. Tension can be a creative force in the organization, but the source of the tension should not be fear but instead a person's motivation to achieve and excel through a positive set of incentives.

Herzberg makes a strong case for job enrichment as a way of motivating people. Job enrichment, he suggests, loads a job vertically, not horizontally. Horizontal loading "merely enlarges the meaninglessness of the job." He suggests that doing 20,000 bolts a day rather than 10,000 or doing two meaningless tasks rather than one is simply of little value. Vertical loading (or enrichment) makes the job more meaningful by giving the employee greater control over the processes and inputs. For example, he suggests "removing some controls while retaining accountability" as one mechanism of motivating people through their own sense of personal responsibility and achievement.

A second mechanism Herzberg suggests is shortening the evaluation and feedback loops by "making periodic reports directly available to the worker himself rather than to the supervisor." This is a way of providing internal recognition. In discussing his ideas, Herzberg clearly states that it is management's responsibility to develop the job enrichment scheme and that the value of employee participation in the development phases is limited. He notes that "it is the content that will produce the motivation, not attitudes about being involved or the challenge inherent in setting up a job." Some jobs in health care lend themselves to job enrichment activities, but others, because of technical or legal requirements, would be excluded as candidates for enrichment.

A different, perhaps related, approach is that of active, effective, or dynamic listening. This is an idea that is found in management communication as well as child development literature. The notion is deceivingly simple: listen to what people really mean when they talk. The problem is that most people communicate in a coded form; to be most responsive, the listener must break through the code. Motivation of another requires a true understanding of what that person is saying and feeling. Thus, a spoken message must be examined on a variety of levels and responded to at the most useful level.

There are also a great many nonverbal messages to which the active listener can respond, e.g., low productivity, absenteeism, poor quality work, and other indicators of a person's distress. Many managers want to be able to rectify these situations with a quick stroke of the pen or a few words; oftentimes, however, a significantly greater investment is necessary before there is any return.

ORGANIZATIONAL MOTIVATION

A related issue is what motivates this impersonal entity called an organization? For example, why would a hospital decide to develop an innovative ambulatory care program? What does such a development mean to management and those people potentially involved with such a program? A hospital usually involves itself in a new ambulatory care program for several reasons. There may be a declining census ("If we had a new ambulatory care program we could assure ourselves of a flow of patients") and a companion problem of finances, which could be helped if a new service were developed to utilize the ancillary services such as laboratory and x-ray. Another problem might be competition from a hospital across the street or across town. The most likely reason for involvement in new programs is some difficulty with existing facilities and programs. Typically, the traffic in the emergency room has increased dramatically with nonemergency patients; staffing is not optimal; follow-up is poor; and the hospital views itself as extremely vulnerable to lawsuits, poor public relations, and poor medical care unless it does something. The something then becomes a new program or a major reorganization.

Other factors that generate a demand for innovation and change include a perceived patient demand for services, which is often verified through a statistical analysis; the need of an institution to fulfill its "destiny" to become a community or comprehensive institution; and, finally, the need of people within the organization to get their own adrenalin flowing through planning and developing new programs.

Assuming that a community hospital has decided to develop an ambulatory care program, what kind of people should it hire for its management and delivery staff? Who should be the medical director, manager, physicians, nurses, and others? Should they be certain kinds of people or will virtually anyone do? It is argued here that, although the motivation of the people who are engaged to begin this project is critical to its initial success, the project's viability over the long run may be related to either the development of the original team or its replacement. Just as football teams have found that they can be most successful with offensive and defensive teams, organizations may have to learn that there are certain people who need the excitement of working in young and developing programs, while others prefer to work in the older, more established programs.

What is needed initially is a group of hardy people who can stand up to the pressure of a medical staff that is likely to be less than enthusiastic, perhaps even hostile, and who thrive on the excitement of moving into uncharted areas. These are people who love the excitement of change and debate and are skilled enough to reach desired outcomes. In some ways, these are the gourmet cooks of the management field. They love trying something new and different; they are very skillful, but the fun is in the cooking (once) and not in the eating. Such persons are motivated by challenge, responsibility, autonomy, and recognition. They are not turned on by security or personal survival.

The organization's time frame and interests go on significantly longer than those of the people involved in developing the program. While the innovators are interested in starting a new and exciting program, the hospital must be concerned about the program's existence in ten years. To keep that first team interested may require continual changes in the new program, changes that are unnecessary or even unacceptable to the hospital. For example, a community hospital develops a hospital-based ambulatory care group practice with four physicians and a manager. It takes two very exciting years to establish this practice, and by the middle of the third year it is running smoothly and breaking even financially. Everyone gives much credit for the success of the program to the group's medical director and manager, who have been involved since the program's inception and have nurtured it since its infancy. The founding fathers are bound together because of the internal developmental problems as well as the external threats they have faced. Listening to them over coffee is like overhearing veterans of the Battle of the Bulge on Friday night at the VFW post. Three years later, the practice has become routine, and the old war horses are ready for some new challenges.

The question for the institution is whether these challenges should come inside the practice (Is change necessary for the practice itself or to keep the staff motivated?) or outside the practice. Is it time for the developmental team to move on and be replaced by others whose motivation is different? The answer is related to what the organization wants to do with that program. If the organization does not wish to take an active stand, then a new round of developments, such as program expansion or facility and staff changes, can be expected. These will inevitably be justified on the basis of patient demand, but, in large part, they may be generated by the developers' need to feed their own motivational needs.

LEADERSHIP AND MANAGEMENT

Is there something called leadership, or is it a euphemism for good management? The literature of management is replete with articles on leadership, formal and informal, and the role that leaders play in organizations. The military and other large organizations often provide training in leadership; yet there is controversy over the very existence of leadership types and management types. Some of the controversy is related to the academic interventions, suggesting that leadership can be taught, much like financial techniques. In fact, in the field of health administration, there is an on-going debate over who shall train the leaders and who shall train the managers. All of this is rather value-laden in that leaders are considered the top level group and managers are at least a rung or two down.

In a superb article on the subject, Zalesnick argues that managers and leaders are different type people.[16] It is recognized, of course, that certain people are leaders by virtue of their positions, such as the director of a community mental health center or a hospital; at a different level, there can be a certain degree of leadership from a department head or supervisor. The critical points that Zalesnick raises concern the type of behavior seen in a leader and the type of behavior seen in a manager. He suggests that managers and leaders differ in attitudes toward goals, conceptions of work, behavior toward risk taking, relations with others, and their sense of self. He suggests that leaders are active in terms of setting goals and tend to personalize them, that is, they see goals as an extension of themselves. Managers' views of goals, on the other hand, are rather impersonal and are directed by the organizational needs. It is suggested that managers respond to goals; they do not initiate them. Their goals do not become the organization's, but rather the organization's goals become theirs. In terms of conceptions of work, leaders are characterized by Zalesnick as movers and shakers, artists who are very much integrated into their own works. They are, he suggests, visionaries—people who excite others with their own vision of what could or should happen. Managers are the doers—those who, through their skills, can make things happen. Everyone has known people who had great ideas but were simply unable to implement them—thus, the simple dichotomy.

This dichotomy, according to Zalesnick, leads to a different type of risk behavior on the part of the two principal types. Leaders like to gamble and take risks—they get excited about the possible return on their enormous investment. Managers are considerably more conservative; they tend to be survival-oriented and are much more calculating, perhaps far more reality-oriented. A leader's concept of reality may be more global and is certainly more challenging than that of the manager.

In terms of working with others, Zalesnick clearly characterizes managers as people who have a need to work with others but in a somewhat orchestrated way. He suggests that managers are role players who might say to themselves, "If I am a manager, what should I do?'' Much of their time and effort is spent in conflict resolutions, which requires them to wear various masks. This might lead people to ask about a manager: "I wonder what kind of person he really is?'' Leaders seem to have more highly charged relationships with others, perhaps love-hate relationships. When they get involved, they get deeply involved. It sometimes appears that leaders have no gray areas in their relationships—they are either on or off.

A final area considered by Zalesnick is that of self-concept. He suggests that leaders feel very much a part of a global community, not simply a part of an organization. Managers derive a major portion of their identity from the organization that employs them, but a leader's identity is very much supraorganization.

Based on the author's research in ambulatory care organization, in which a few dozen of these developing and established programs were studied, it appears that such personality types do indeed exist and are important to organizations. For example, several years ago, a 400-bed hospital located in a major metropolitan area received a modest grant from a private foundation to start a hospital-based ambulatory care unit. It engaged as its program director a 40-year-old physician who was trained as a surgeon but wished to work full-time for the institution to start this program and to organize all their ambulatory care facilities. He was an exciting and attractive person who seemed to inspire very strong feelings (both positive and negative) on the part of those he met. His vision of ambulatory care was very much in concert with that of the foundation, the hospital director, and the board, but quite contrary to that of the hospital medical staff. Over the first year of the new program, he spent much of his time sharing his vision and convincing the medical staff of its accuracy. He was interested only in the broad outlines of making the program functional, not the details. His friends and adversaries described him as a charmer, a diplomat, a hip shooter. His ideas and plans were rarely carefully detailed but always exciting. His personnel decisions tended to be made quickly, seemingly by instinct. For example, a young physician in the program had been with this man only a few minutes when he was offered the job. The director liked him and that was enough.

Managing the program was a 30-year-old business school graduate. Rarely was he involved in generating major new concepts for change, but he was in a sense the leader's simultaneous translator, taking his ideas and visions, perhaps putting a bit of his own personal twist on it, and then translating these concepts into a workable plan. The manager enjoyed understanding which buttons to push to make the program function and then pushing the buttons.

Both of these people were most excited by the idea of working in a new, innovative, and somewhat glamorous program. As the program started to age, however, each became a bit disenchanted, not by the program but by the lack of managerial challenge for one and the lack of leadership challenge for the other. The leader went off to take on new tasks and become more involved in activities outside the hospital. The manager, on the other hand, looked within the job for more challenges and eventually began searching for a new and more challenging managerial position.

In this example, the two people recognized themselves and each other as a manager and a leader, and they were pleased to be playing their respective roles. They enjoyed each other's professional company and respected each other, although they were totally uninvolved socially and knew little about each other's lives outside of the institution. They were in every sense of the word a team that worked. While it was important for the manager to recognize and not be threatened by the presence of a strong leader, it was equally important for the leader to recognize that his ideas and programs would be so much hot air unless a manager translated them into action programs. The hospital administrators had not planned this strategy of organization, but, having observed its functioning, they have become extremely sensitized to its value.

How does an organization recognize people who are motivated in one way or another? This is a chemistry problem, since how people react and function in one organization may not indicate how they will behave in a different situation. Universities are often confronted by applicants who have had poor undergraduate records and now want to go to graduate school. They always say that they were not motivated before. What has happened between 18 and 21 that may turn a mediocre undergraduate student into a star graduate student? The answer, it would appear, has to do with the chemistry of maturity and ambition—the person is now "turned on." While one clear indicator of probable success is a person's track record, others might be evident to someone who is listening carefully to an applicant. The challenge then to management is not only to recognize obvious talent but also to "turn on" latent talent.

CASE STUDY

Hospital Housekeeping Care

The housekeeping department at the 330-bed Jewish Hospital of Philadelphia is managed by Mrs. Ethel Greenburg, a 55-year-old widow who is a Russian immigrant. Prior to working at this hospital, Mrs. Greenburg spent eight years as the assistant executive housekeeper at Central General Hospital in Philadelphia, a 550-bed government hospital. Mrs. Greenburg's background includes one year of nurse's training in Moscow, and graduation from a two-year post-high-school training program at the Soviet National School of Hotel Management in Moscow. In the Soviet Union, Mrs. Greenburg worked in various administrative capacities in different hotels. Prior to leaving her country, she was one of four assistant managers at a 300-room modern "intercontinental" hotel. Since arriving in the United States ten years ago, Mrs. Greenburg has been active in hospital housekeeping circles, attending seminars and professional meetings.

In Mrs. Greenburg's present assignment as executive housekeeper of Jewish Hospital of Philadelphia, she is responsible for a staff of 20 men and 25 women, as well as for the administration of a budget of $750,000. Approximately half of the employees in the department are Hispanics, and the other half are Blacks, including several from Haiti. The department is organized with Mrs. Greenburg as the head and Mr. Iglesiada, a Puerto Rican, as assistant head. All staff assignments are approved by Mrs. Greenburg weekly after Mr. Iglesiada submits to her a schedule of activities for each cleaner, maid, and janitor. Both Mrs. Greenburg and Mr. Iglesiada interview each prospective employee. Mr. Iglesiada has been at the hospital for nine years and has worked his way up from janitor to assistant department head. Prior to Mrs. Greenburg's arrival, he functioned adequately as acting department head for three months. The previous department head retired from the position after 37 years at the hospital. He was generally well regarded by the employees but viewed as unprofessional and a poor manager by the management.

Since Mrs. Greenburg's arrival, the quality of housekeeping in the institution has improved slightly; relations between the department heads of housekeeping, dietary, laundry, maintenance, and nursing have become markedly better, but the morale among the staff has deteriorated. Turnover and absenteeism have increased dramatically, and it appears that union activity has increased in this unit.

Ths assistant administrator has discussed the morale problem with Mrs. Greenburg, who feels that Mr. Iglesiada is undermining her efforts to professionalize the housekeeping service. Mr. Iglesiada, she contends, is making it difficult to install new mechanized cleaning equipment, develop more efficient work schedules, and run an effective inservice training program. Mrs. Greenburg's analysis is that the department had been loosely run and that treatment based on favoritism had been the norm under the previous department head.

Mr. Iglesiada argues that Mrs. Greenburg was a bad choice for the job because she is insensitive to the needs of the workers and is only interested in "her own ego trip," not the best interests of the hospital. Mr. Iglesiada has threatened to quit unless Mrs. Greenburg is dismissed—and he says that half the department will leave if he does.

The assistant administrator thinks that, if Mr. Iglesiada left, about 10 or 15 employees might also quit. Also, although he believes that Mr. Iglesiada did an adequate job as acting department head, he does not have the managerial experience and perhaps the potential (although there is uncertainty about this) to be the department head.

Discussion Questions

1. What are the probable points of conflict between Mrs. Greenburg and Mr. Iglesiada? Between Mrs. Greenburg and the staff?
2. What options are available for resolution? What might be the costs and benefits of these optional resolutions?

NOTES

1. C.P. McCormick, *The Power of People* (Baltimore: produced for McCormick by Penguin Books, 1949).
2. R.T. LaPierre, "Attitudes vs. Actions," *Social Forces* 13 (1934):230-237.
3. L.G. Warner, and M.E. DeFleur, "Attitude as an Interactional Concept: Social Constraint and Social Distance as Intervening Variables Between Attitudes and Action," *American Sociological Review* 34, no. 2 (April 1969):153-169.
4. A. Maslow, *Motivation and Personality* (New York: Harper & Row, 1954), pp. 80-106.
5. A. Maslow, *Eupsychian Management* (Homewood, IL: Irwin-Dorsey, 1965).
6. F. Herzberg, "One More Time—How Do You Motivate Employees?" *Harvard Business Review*" 46 (Jan-Feb 1968):1, 53-82.
7. Douglas McGregor, "The Human Side of Enterprise" in *Management of Human Resources*, ed. by P. Pigois, C.A. Myers, and F.T. Malm (New York: McGraw-Hill, 1964), pp. 55-61.
8. P.F. Drucker, *Management* (New York: Harper & Row, 1974), p. 233.
9. A.M. Carr-Sanders and P.A. Wilson, *The Professions* (Oxford: Clarendon Press, 1933), p. 284.
10. *Aulen v. Triumph Explosive* D.C. Md. 58 F. Supp. 4.
11. S. Bloom, *The Doctor and His Patient* (New York: The Free Press, 1965), p. 89.
12. D.R. Hyde et al, *Yale Law Journal* 63(1954):7, pp. 937-1022.
13. R.A. Kessel, "Price Discrimination in Medicine," *Journal of Law and Economics* I (1958):2, pp. 20-53.
14. T. Parsons, *The Social System* (Glencoe, IL: The Free Press, 1961), pp. 428-460.
15. J. Heller, *Something Happened* (New York: Ballantine, 1975), p. 9.
16. A. Zalesnick, "Managers and Leaders: Are They Different?" *Harvard Business Review* 55, no. 3 (May-June 1977), pp. 67-78.

Chapter 8

Machiavelli and Health Care Management

The essential element in the practice of health administration is politics. The notion that a health administrator's job is political strikes some as simply abhorrent, but it is also realistic. Administrators are continually called upon to allocate scarce resources among competing factions and simultaneously to maintain something akin to an equilibrium in the organization. To do this requires the political skills of persuasion, knowledge, and empathy. Also, administrators must be relatively secure in what they are doing and clear as to their goals.

Perhaps the single greatest text written on politics, which can certainly offer numerous lessons for health administration, was the early sixteenth-century work by Niccolò Machiavelli. Machiavelli wrote *The Prince*[1] as a gift for Lorenzo de Medici in order to help the Florentine ruler understand the politics of management and leadership. Machiavelli viewed management and leadership in an almost amoral way, and his purpose in preparing his text was to curry favor with those in power so that he could reattain a governmental position from which he had been dismissed after an apparently successful career as a senior level official.

PHASE I—THE MANAGEMENT HONEYMOON

One of the first sections in *The Prince* is titled "Composite Principalities." In that chapter Machiavelli writes of the problems likely to be experienced by a new monarch. He begins by noting the fickleness of people; he suggests that, because people's expectations are not usually met, they are always willing to accept a different leader. Other points that Machiavelli makes include the importance of obtaining and maintaining the good will of the people in the new country and identifying allies and potential enemies, such as members of the deposed family. In this, as well as elsewhere, Machiavelli suggests that those who oppose must be eliminated.

A few of his major points have particular relevance to health administration, since administrators are often taking someone else's job (at least it is perceived in that way). Sometimes the person who is leaving or has left has voluntarily resigned and is leaving with all good thoughts on everyone's part; other times the resignation has been requested, and there is ill will throughout the organization. The former incumbent has supporters and detractors. The supporters feel they lost; the detractors smell a victory. The new administrator has probably not been involved in the battles but is immediately asked to choose sides.

This phenomenon was illustrated at a rural New Jersey hospital where, within a few weeks of his arrival, a new chief executive officer was challenged by the medical staff on a basic issue that related to the special organization of this institution (it was a closed-staff fee-for-service institution). His response, however justified, recreated the tension that had been smoldering since the resignation of the former chief executive officer and redrew the battle lines that had existed. This fight, while inevitable, came at a most inopportune time for the new administrator: before he was able to identify his allies and likely protagonists, and before he was able to establish his own power base. In essence, he was forced to do battle without the proper support lines, and the net result was that he was forced to resign within a few months.

Machiavelli suggests that it is critical that the new "ruler" establish his territoriality. He must let everyone know that he is in fact the new ruler, by words and deeds. At the simplest and most superficial level, he must move into his new office and make that office state that he is there and that it is his. One manager accepted an important position at a large teaching hospital, but part of the agreement with the institution was that he could be away two days a week on consulting work. For the three years he was there, his office always looked vacant: a big desk, a table and chairs, and bookshelves. It looked almost like a Madison Avenue showroom rather than a line manager's office. This manager was sending messages to those around him that his heart and soul were elsewhere. His effectiveness was also diminished because, although most people he encountered admired his intelligence and judgment, none took him seriously and thus they easily stonewalled his programs. Even his supporters were reluctant to pit themselves against his detractors; after all, it was reasoned that he would not be there in a year or two to take the heat. And they were right.

A good example of how managers establish territoriality can be found in the military. During the five years that I was a naval officer, I served under five commanding officers, and each one of them held an inspection on Friday mornings. The inspection was usually rather informal, but virtually every nook and cranny of the hospital was inspected by the commanding officer and his entourage. These inspections also included verbal interchanges (usually pleasant) between the commanding officer and whoever was present, including patients on the ward. Most of the commanding officers used the time to see for themselves what was going on and to make themselves accessible to the staff. For example, one always had his scribe keep a list of the problems that had been identified on inspection. On subsequent inspections, he would follow up to ascertain the problem's resolution. On the psychological level, the commanding officer was saying that he was indeed responsible for (and to a degree had the authority to change) what was going on in the institution.

It is interesting to note how few executives personally make their presence felt in an institution. In many ways it is more secure and certainly easier to stay in an office. This even happens in university administration. For example, there was a professor at a school of public health who in over a year had never met the new dean. After four years in office, a vice chancellor had never visited one of the three constituent schools of his chancellorship, despite the fact that the school was less than a block away and his relationship with its staff was positive.

When Machiavelli suggests that "one of the best, most effective expedients would be for the conqueror to go to live there in person," he is giving important advice on establishing territoriality and managerial presence, another thing accomplished by the weekly inspections. Such a presence allows subordinates to feel comfortable in the knowledge (or at least belief) that there is someone at a higher level who is capable of making decisions, and it allows for maintenance of the organization. Machiavelli notes these points:

> Being on the spot, one can detect trouble at the start and deal with it immediately; if one is absent, it is discerned only when it has grown serious, and it is then too late. And besides, this policy prevents the conquered territory from being plundered by one's officials. The subjects are satisfied because they have direct recourse to the prince. . . .

Being there and being accessible, then, are two points of importance. The military inspection can be translated into administrative rounds, and presence into literally being there. In other words, managers should take one job, not two. They should work for one organization, not two. They should be evaluated by one boss, not two. A novel way one hospital administrator handles the presence issue is through a "zone defense." He does this by assigning each of the front office subordinates to a physically different section of the hospital. In this way, virtually everyone in the institution has easy access to a front office administrator and, according to the hospital director, problems are spotted early and resolved before they get out of hand.

The final advice from Machiavelli in the third chapter is that the prince must be a a wise planner:

> . . . the Romans did what all wise rulers must: cope not only with present troubles but with ones likely to arise in the future, and assidu-

ously forestall them. When trouble is sensed well in advance it can be easily remedied; if you wait for it to show itself any medicine will be too late because the disease will become incurable.

The wise manager, Machiavelli would suggest, is a wise planner. He is organizing and husbanding his time and resources and is waiting for the right moment. A former senior executive in government once said that, when he was in Washington, he had a file drawer full of future plans and that his effectiveness was in large part related to the quality of his plans, coupled with the correctness of his timing. Effectiveness, he suggested, was having the right plan or solution available at the right time.

PHASE II—CONSOLIDATION

In Chapter 4, in which he discusses why the kingdom of Darius conquered by Alexander did not rebel against his successors after his death, and Chapter 5, how cities or principalities which lived under their own laws should be administered after being conquered, Machiavelli suggests alternative managerial approaches. Using the Turkish and French Empires as examples, he contrasts centralized and decentralized power. He suggests that a kingdom, such as Turkey, with a centralized power system where everyone is responsible to the king and all authority is exercised by him or his agents at his direction, would be difficult to conquer. Once conquered, however, it would be easy to administer because one strong man would be substituted for another, and people were used to a central authority. This is contrasted with the decentralized form in France where there was "a long established order of nobles, who are acknowledged in France by their own subjects and are loved by them. They have their prerogatives; the king cannot take these away from them except at his own peril."

In Chapter 5, Machiavelli reiterates his advice concerning what the conqueror should do in order to maintain his new kingdom:

When states newly acquired, as I said, have been accustomed to living freely under their own laws, there are three ways to hold them securely: first, by devastating them; next, by going and living there in person; thirdly, by letting them keep their own laws, exacting tribute, and setting up an oligarchy which will keep the state friendly to you.

Clearly, Machiavelli came down on the side of options three and two, and not in favor of one.

His arguments for centralization and decentralization in a sense strike at the core issue—power. To what degree can management feel secure if people who are essentially subordinates have independent power? The centralized mode is quite clearly a replication of the paternalistic (or maternalistic) family—one person is effectively a benevolent dictator. Decentralization seems to have not only the greatest dispersion of power but also the most stable power base.

In health care organizations, two phenomena can be observed: (1) there is an uncontrollable decentralization of power and authority to the professional staff, and (2) there is often a high labor turnover at the top and bottom levels of the organization and great stability in the middle. For example, in one large municipal hospital in the South, top management was totally immersed in state health care (and other) politics and was certainly not attending to the problems of this large teaching hospital. This operation managed to function because there had been a significant decentralization of authority and responsibility that had resulted in a strong and solid middle management capable of carrying on despite the climate at the top.

PHASE III—LOYALTY AND INNOVATION

Loyalty, to Machiavelli, is one of the key elements in the success of a new manager or leader. Loyalty that runs deep would more likely be generated by Theory Y behavior and attitudes than those of Theory X. Loyalty is earned, Machiavelli suggests. Care must be taken not to confuse acquiescence for loyalty. Perhaps one of the most difficult jobs of a manager, particularly one new to a job, is to avoid the clever sycophant.

As noted earlier, one of the important strategies that management can adopt is that of innovation—fostering it and being innovative itself. On the subject of innovation, Machiavelli notes in Chapter 6 (New principalities acquired by one's own arms and prowess):

> The innovator makes enemies of all those who prospered under the old order, and only lukewarm support is forthcoming from those who would prosper under the new. Their support is lukewarm partly from fear of their adversaries, who have the existing laws on their side and partly because men are generally incredulous, never really trusting new things unless they have tested them by experience. In consequence, whenever those who oppose the changes can do so, they attack vigorously, and the defense made by the others is only lukewarm. So both the innovator and his friends are endangered together . . . all armed prophets have conquered and unarmed protests have come to grief . . . the populace is by nature fickle; it is easy to persuade them of something, but difficult to confirm them in that persuasion.

Throughout *The Prince,* Machiavelli appears to admire change, but in this chapter he notes its danger, the principal problem being the inertia and fear of change of those people likely to be affected by the change. Managers, particularly a manager who is new to an organization, are often tempted to use change either as a way of learning how the organization functions, much as a chemist in a laboratory uses tracer elements, or as a way of establishing their territoriality. Both of these reasons are less than optimal approaches to change. It is postulated that any organization can absorb innovation at some rate (not quite clearly determined) and that, when this rate is exceeded, stress in the organization becomes greater than the potential benefit of the innovation. This is somewhat analogous to the capacity of a body of land to retain water; when the absorption rate is exceeded, there are puddles, then pools, and finally a flood.

Another organizational response, equally unsatisfying, occurs when innovations become so commonplace that the workers become inured to them and stonewall them by noncompliance. Since the innovations come so frequently, it is almost impossible to follow up. One hospital administrator commented, "Be careful not to offer more than one new idea a week." A former commissioner in the New York City Department of Hospitals wryly noted one day that he could have the best idea in the world but some "damn grade 2 clerk is simply not going to implement it, and that's the end of my great idea."

Certain types of health care organizations, such as hospitals, are continually bombarded by technical innovations; other types, particularly in the federal government, are always being streamlined by organizational innovations. Innovations, while extremely important, extract a price from any staff, and a staff must be sold on the importance of an innovation before they are likely to cooperate willingly. Machiavelli's description of "armed and unarmed prophets" may be a managerial metaphor for people who have thoroughly researched their ideas and have developed a sound strategy for innovation as opposed to those who come in with half-baked ideas. Since there is a limited absorption rate, managers must take care not to use their innovation bullets carelessly. The unemployment line is filled with former executives who pushed their organizations too fast through the barrier of change. Change is a process that requires intelligence, maturity, and, the most difficult ingredient for an active and fertile innovator, patience.

PHASE IV—DEALING WITH CHALLENGES

In Chapter 6 and in the subsequent three chapters, Machiavelli advises courses of action for those who come to power in different ways: (1) by means of their own strength and wits, (2) with the aid of wealthy and powerful friends, (3) by crime, and (4) by constitutional principles. Analogies can be found in the field of health care management. A new health care administrator may have acquired the position as a result of the death or retirement of the previous beloved administrator. Or, the previous administrator may have been forced to resign by the board after they somewhat reluctantly concluded that he was not terribly competent, although everyone agreed that he was a wonderful person. A third scenario might be that of an administrator who was quite good but was fired because of hostility from the medical staff.

In the first instance, Machiavelli would advise that "a prudent man should always follow in the footsteps of great men and imitate those who have been outstanding." The rationale here is apparently that, if the new administrator can establish linkages to a beloved predecessor, the latter's reservoir of good will can be transferred to the new administrator. The director of a large metropolitan teaching hospital had an 18" × 20" color photograph of the previous administrator on his office wall opposite the couch (where most visitors were likely to sit). The picture was inscribed, "Best personal regards and wishes for success." When asked why he had that, since in private he had made somewhat disparaging comments about his predecessor's ability, the new administrator replied that the man had been helpful to his career and had been much loved in the medical center. Obviously, the photograph was a symbolic link to the past to benefit the present and perhaps the future. The problem for the administrator in this first situation is to acquire the loyalty and devotion that the first one had.

The second administrator is in a somewhat more complicated situation, since the group in power has recognized the incompetence of the administrator but has not acknowledged it publicly. It will be difficult for the new administrator to point out the shortcomings of the well-liked former administrator without offending those in power, who have avoided doing that themselves, or those who supported the former administrator. The problem, Machiavelli would suggest, is that the new administrator has no strong roots in the organization, nor are the roots that are available worthy of transfer: "Governments set up overnight, like everything in nature whose growth is forced, lack strong roots and ramifications. So they are destroyed in the first bad spell." A second and related point that Machiavelli makes is that new administrators do not have any loyalists—people who can be counted on to do the job. Thus, it is imperative that a new administrator approach the job judiciously, taking time to learn about the organization and to understand its history and the nature of the relationships in the organization. Only then will the new administrator become effective in designing and implementing programs and begin to earn loyalty and develop a power base for subsequent operations. In a sense, then, in this example, the new administrator can eventually be accepted as the organizational choice for the management and leadership position. The payoff in such situations, as Machiavelli describes it, is most attractive:

. . . A prince who builds his power on the people, one who can command and is a man of courage, who does not despair in adversity, who does not fail to take precautions, and who wins general allegiance by his personal qualities and the institutions he establishes, he will never be let down by the people; and he will be found to have established his power securely.

In the final example, an administrator who has been enfranchised after the overthrow of the previous one by the power block of the medical staff has some obvious problems. The new administrator is to some extent beholden to the medical staff, who are now feeling their power. To put it another way, the new administrator must appear to be acceptable to this group. The second problem is that many people in the organization have loyalties to the previous administrator, feel that this person was done a grave injustice, and see the new administrator as the manifestation of that injustice. Machiavelli would probably consider this type of situation as the acquisition of power through the crime of others. Although not a participant, the new administrator is certainly the beneficiary of the crime. The advantage in this situation is that, since some blood has been spilled, it is relatively easy to identify the factions and who is likely to be in which camp.

Machiavelli's advice in this instance has earned him his tainted reputation:

> So it should be noted that when he seizes a state the new ruler ought to determine all the injuries that he will need to inflict. He should inflict them once for all, and not have to renew them every day, and in that way he will be able to set men's minds at rest and win them over to him when he confers benefits. Whoever acts otherwise either through timidity or bad advice is always forced to have the knife ready in his hand and he can never depend on his subjects because they, suffering fresh and continuous violence, can never feel secure with regard to him. Violence should be inflicted once for all; people will then forget what it tastes like and so be less resentful. Benefits should be conferred gradually and in that way they will taste better. Above all, a prince should live with his subjects in such a way that no development, either favourable or adverse, makes him vary his conduct. For, when adversity brings the need for it, there is no time to inflict harm; and the favours he may confer are profitless, because they are seen as being forced, and so they earn no thanks.

While this may seem a bit cruel, it does make some pragmatic sense for the new administrator. Firing those people who have to be fired as rapidly as possible is not only politically expedient but also allows the new administrator to build a team that is loyal to him or her. In government, it has long been accepted that, when an administration becomes a lame duck, either by losing an election or by declaring an intention not to run, those on the staff are immediately on the market. Machiavelli is certainly a believer in the notion that to the victors belong the spoils. Management may not be a warlike situation, but it is clearly often a politically active situation, and administrators cannot have people in their camp who are attempting to undermine them or their efforts. In terms of doling out favors, be they programs, money, or stature in the organization, Machiavelli would suggest that the administrator would be wise to dispense favors for a slow and deliberate effect. Again, politicians can be observed doing this; they are servicing their accounts. They are using whatever authority they have to build a strong constituency for their programs. In essence, politicians and administrators are in similar positions; both are in part dependent on quid pro quo relationships for their power.

PHASE V—STRATEGIC PLANNING

Strategic planning is a continuous thread of Machiavelli's philosophy and is of critical importance to any administrator. In Chapter 14 (How a prince should organize his militia) Machiavelli notes that "a wise prince should observe these rules: he should never take things easy in times of peace, but rather use the latter assiduously, in order to be able to reap the profit in time of adversity. Then when his fortunes change he will be found ready to resist adversity." Such notions of planning can be found in a great deal of literature, e.g., the Bible, when Joseph advises Pharoah about the years of a bountiful harvest and the years of famine, and contemporary management texts.

Health administrators spend so much of their energy fighting the crisis of the day that it almost seems there are never times of peace. Indeed there are, but it is sometimes hard to recognize them when the organization and the manager's personal energy system are geared up all the time for full battle. Machiavelli's words could be translated for our purposes by saying that managers must attempt to organize their time so that there are times of peace even in the middle of adversity. Thinking and planning time are precious commodities. People with administrative inclinations are easily seduced into almost hyperactive behavior. Rarely is there a sense of calmness and tranquility in a manager's office. Phones are ringing, people popping in and out, intercoms buzzing, and schedules that begin early in the morning go late into the evening. It is indeed very ego-satisfying to be "desired" by so many people, but the question remains: what kind of planning/thinking time is available and to what extent is such an executive developing the means to prevent executive burnout?

Fire-fighting is the present; strategic planning is the future, and most of what happens to an organization will happen in the future. Good planning will over time minimize the fire-fighting and certainly mitigate its potential destructiveness. A commitment for administrators to allow themselves the private time for planning and reflection is too often viewed as a luxury rather than a necessity, however. In Chapter 17 of *The Prince,* Machiavelli talks of cruelty and compassion, and whether it is better to be loved or feared. He proposes that a prince should want to have "a reputation for compassion rather than cruelty; nonetheless, he should be careful that he does not make bad use of compassion." He goes on to distinguish between different degrees of compassion, arguing that too much compassion results in anarchy, which works to the detriment of the entire community, while appropriate compassion occasionally affects individuals negatively but has an overall positive effect on the community.

The administrator who wants to be loved and says "yes" to everyone about everything is assuming that this is the path to credibility and respect. Indeed, it is actually a path in the opposite direction. Administrators are paid to make tough resource allocation decisions. In a fair percentage of these decisions, the administrator has considerable latitude, and this is where compassion can and should be exercised.

Sometimes, a decision may be "cruel" to an individual and yet most compassionate in terms of the work community. For example, what should be done with an offensive and obnoxious worker who is disrupting the work of others and who obviously has serious psychological problems? The most compassionate solution for the individual may be the least compassionate for the group. Balancing these conflicting needs, as well as the administrator's personal needs, is a difficult process with no clear-cut and totally satisfactory solutions.

In the next chapter (How princes should honor their words), Machiavelli provides considerable food for thought. Basically, he makes the case that the means justify the ends, that situational ethics prevail, and that image is at least as important (and maybe more so) as substance:

> Princes who have achieved great things have been those who have given their word lightly, who have known how to trick men with their cunning, and who, in the end, have overcome those abiding by honest principles . . . a prudent ruler cannot, and should not, honour his word when it places him at a disadvantage and when the reasons for which he has made his promise no longer exist. If all men were good, this precept would not be good; but because men are wretched creatures who would not keep their word to you, you need not keep your word to them.

Obviously, Machiavelli is a Theory X man. He does not trust people and views them as fickle, at best. "Men are so simple, and so much creatures of circumstance, that the deceiver will always find someone ready to be deceived."

In discussing image and substance, Machiavelli points out that to those "seeing and hearing him [the prince] he should appear a man of compassion, a man of good faith, a man of integrity, a kind and religious man. . . ." Machiavelli then offers this advice, "So let a prince set about the task of conquering and maintaining his state; his methods will always be judged honourable and will be universally

praised. The common people are always impressed by appearances and results."
Like the emperor in the children's fairy tale, *The Emperor's New Clothes,* the
prince can always be assured that those around him and those dependent on his
good will (and good humor) will not want to be the messenger with the bad news.
Indeed, in the recent studies of the presidency there have been numerous examples
of senior staff and even cabinet level people who have skewed their observations
and analyses to please the president and distort reality.

The issue of means and ends is a very sensitive one in the health care establishment, in part because of the large number of voluntary boards that have considerable authority but limited involvement in implementation. In one case, the chairman of a hospital's board had a reputation in philanthropic and business circles as
an unethical person and, for that reason, had found it difficult to get on a hospital
board. The one that did accept him promptly elevated him to a very high position
because of small gifts and the promise of larger ones. Is it appropriate for an
institution to honor someone who is less than honorable? Is the legitimacy of the
institution and its board for sale?

Machiavelli would argue that the benefits would clearly outweigh the costs. In
the aforementioned example, it should be pointed out that the involvement of this
person in an important post on the board probably repelled others, some of whom
may have been of more value in a variety of ways. This person never gave the
hospital any sizable amount of money, and he used the hospital as a means of
dealing with his own personal and business frustrations. For example, when the
hospital was in the early stages of unionization, he directed an all-out offensive
against the union, which included physical violence. Why the massive response?
A large part of the reason seems to have been the fact that his own business—and
he himself in the bargain—was on several occasions brought to its knees by a
powerful union. In his plants, he was continually waging a losing battle with the
union; in fact, the National Labor Relations Board had made decisions against him
and his firm for serious unfair labor practices. Under this man's influence, the
hospital's response to its union was not related to the issues but rather to its board
chairman's overall anger toward unions. Obviously, he lived his life, as the
institution and its management did, with the notion that the ends justified the
means. Thus, the price paid by the hospital may have far exceeded any immediate
or potential long-range benefit of having this person as chairman of their board.
Regardless, the ethical fiber of the institution was clearly weakened by this
person's presence.

In the next two chapters of *The Prince* (The need to avoid contempt and hatred
and Whether fortresses and many other present day expedients to which princes
have recourse are useful or not), Machiavelli suggests some interesting concepts
about interpersonal relationships. He begins by noting that, if people are angry
with or hate the prince, he must always be afraid of everything and everyone. On
the other hand, he suggests that "well organized states and wise princes have

always taken great pains not to make nobles despair, and to satisfy the people and keep them content."

To effect this, Machiavelli suggests several strategies. First, he suggests that unpopular acts should be delegated to others while the prince should always be the one who passes out favors. Some administrators, however, seem to thrive on tension and adversity. Indeed, one successful executive took great pleasure in searching for assistant administrators who had what he described as the killer instinct.

A second problem Machiavelli identifies is that of satisfying multiple (and in many cases irreconcilable) constituencies. In *The Prince,* Machiavelli uses the example of a new ruler trying simultaneously to appease war-loving soldiers and the peace-loving populace. The administrator of a health care organization must recognize that perhaps dozens of constituencies must be dealt with, and each one is motivated in a different way. Sometimes meeting the demands of one constituency would offend another. The solution, according to Machiavelli, is to "strive assiduously to escape the hatred of the most powerful classes." Good advice—but sometimes it is difficult to tell which group is most powerful, which group will become most powerful later, and, finally, how power and correctness can be reconciled on a given issue.

Next, Machiavelli returns to the importance of image. He suggests that the downfall of one Roman ruler was related to an image problem. "He forgot his dignity, often descended into the amphitheaters to fight with the gladiators, and did other ignoble things hardly worthy of the imperial majesty; as a result the soldiers came to despise him."

This then leads Machiavelli to a prescription for success. First, he notes that the prince must build a staff loyal to himself; this is in part accomplished by arming people:

> Those who were suspect become loyal, and those who were loyal not only remain so but are changed from being merely your subjects to being your partisans.

Then he suggests having these people engage in a few "battles" where their victory is assured to build a sense of confidence and esprit de corps. Finally, he proposes that the prince must keep his people busy with worthwhile projects. Machiavelli seems to agree with the saying that "idle hands are the devil's workshop."

Machiavelli's proposals here appear to make considerable sense in health administration. Invest in people, develop them, and they will provide a good return for that investment. Keep them busy on serious and worthwhile projects, praise them in public, damn them in private—help people feel confident about themselves. The philosophy expressed in these sections of Machiavelli is similar to that of Drucker who emphasizes the importance of management development.[2]

The next two chapters of *The Prince* (A prince's personal staff and How flatterers must be shunned) are really the key to Machiavelli's thinking. Of course, they are written out of Machiavelli's self-interest because he wished to ingratiate himself with Lorenzo and thereby earn a position in his administraton. He points out that the most important decisions are those made about the prince's senior staff:

> The first opinion that is formed of a ruler's intelligence is based on the quality of the men he has around him. When they are competent and loyal he can always be considered wise, because he has been able to recognize their competence and keep them loyal. But when they are otherwise, the prince is always open to adverse criticism, because his first mistake has been in the choice of ministers.

Machiavelli advises looking for deputies who can "understand things for itself"—a second level person would be one who "appreciates what others can understand." To be avoided is someone with little capacity for understanding.

A caution he raises is that noted earlier about sycophants; he suggests that top aides should understand that the prince values the "truth" but that the prince sets the time and tone of the truth. In essence, he argues that universal access to the prince denigrates his role and power. Thus, the prince should select who shall talk to him on what matters, but the staff must know that the prince expects and values truth.

These final lessons about senior staff are quite relevant in the health industry where recruiting decisions are oftentimes made in a most thoughtless and cavalier way. While most organizations can carry out a competent executive search without consultants, it is nevertheless interesting to note how poorly recruiting is done in large segments of the health field. Indeed, as Machiavelli suggests, the most important decisions to be made are those about recruiting—they have ramifications that could make or break an organization or program.

In the concluding sections of his volume, Machiavelli notes that, despite all good warnings and plans, sometimes environmental factors, over which the prince has quite limited control, conspire against him and his plans go astray.

It may be asked whether any of Machiavelli's assertions have direct relevance to the operational problems of today's health care organization. What advice would Machiavelli give regarding an innovative hospital-based ambulatory care program that has been developed over the objections of a medical staff and perhaps a few trustees? He would probably say that a constituency should be developed for the program. This constituency might be a loose coalition of patients, staff, and physicians. The constituency could be built by services offered, interpersonal relations, personal diplomacy, organizational relations (e.g., staff conferences or participative management), and public relations activities such as newsletters and tours.

Secondly, he would say that enemies should be identified and neutralized. At one level, if the manager were powerful enough, enemies might be isolated, i.e., excluded from the hospital. More commonly, innovators attempt to demonstrate that they are not a threat but can be helpful. In one situation, two physicians hostile to the program were neutralized in a way that was beneficial to both the physicians and their practice. In one case, the physician was retiring, and the hospital arranged to buy his practice; in the second case, the physician wished to go into semiretirement and the hospital brought his patients into the group and hired him on a part-time basis. These former opponents became the most important supporters of the program.

Next, Machiavelli would advise continual vigilance to what is happening in the environment and what the "competition" is doing. Strategic planning is critical even for a small hospital-based group practice in these unsettled times. Finally, Machiavelli would suggest recruiting managers, leaders, and practitioners in order to succeed.

In sum, Machiavelli provides a good lesson in the "realpolitik" of complex organizations. Some of his ideas and concepts are, to say the least, distasteful; however, many are extremely useful to present day health care management.

NOTES

1. N. Machiavelli, *The Prince* (New York: Penguin, 1975).
2. P.F. Drucker, *Management* (New York: Harper & Row, 1974), pp. 419-429.

Chapter 9

Structure and Staffing of Health Care Organizations

All organizations have a structure—sometimes that structure is shown on an organization chart; other times the structure is unclear on first inspection. Regardless of the presumed structure, there are two major points to keep in mind. First, there is no magic in any given structure. A well-structured organization is no guarantee of success. A corollary of this point is that no structure is sacrosanct. A structure that may work at one time might not work at a later time. The second major point is that a structure is similar to a roadmap; it gives an observer an idea about relationships and distance, but it does not provide an in-depth understanding of power, personalities, or functions.

Why bother to have an organizational structure? In one sense, there is an easy answer—it is unavoidable. Whether or not the structure is committed to a piece of paper and labeled an organization chart, the organization has a structure. At the simplest level, there is the one-person organization where all authority and responsibility are vested in a single individual. When the organization increases its size by 100 percent to two persons, some structure must be developed; otherwise, duplication of activities and perhaps conflict result. Functions, responsibility, and authority must be delineated and assigned. As the organization expands and more staff are hired, more structure is imposed—and each step of structural development requires a clearer definition of organizational goals, responsibility, and authority. Structure then is a shorthand for identifying significant relationships. To a limited extent, it also provides information about the processes in the organizations.

People are socialized to organizational structure practically from birth. In families, parents serve as the top managers; there is division of labor, some delegation of responsibility, and, no doubt, conflict. Nursery schools, grade schools, and virtually any job introduce structured organizations.

135

The structure itself sets up certain expectations. For example, in a classic pyramid structure there is one person on top. Two people report to this person, several people report to these two people, and so forth. It is expected that communication up or down the organization will go through the specified chain of command. This is how the military functions, and going outside the chain is considered unacceptable organizational behavior. Thus, while a Navy Captain or sailor, as citizens of the United States, have the right to correspond with their senator or representative, it would be frowned upon for either of these people to go to their elected official to register a complaint about how something was functioning in the naval service. Their recourse, it would be argued, is the next step up the chain of command, and going to Congress would be jumping too many levels on the chain.

A final point on the notion of expectations is that the pyramid structure provides many people with a strong sense of security. It lets them know to whom they are responsible and for whom they are responsible; it tells them something about the path they must follow to reach any personal or professional goals. In organizations where this is unclear, it appears that individuals with a strong sense of personal direction are able to climb the illusory ladder faster than people who need greater direction and tend to get stymied.

Most other organizational forms are simply variations on the pyramid. Recently, there has been more discussion about the ruling junta approach—the office of the chief executive route. In this structure, a team at the top runs the organization, and teams may function at lower levels. Clearly though, team members have their own strengths and weaknesses, and thus the teams to some extent become pyramidal in a functional sense.

The matrix organization is a variation of the team approach. A type of cooperative relationship is developed between the vertical and horizontal hierarchies involved in a particular function. For example, a typical hospital patient floor has people working from several different departmental areas, and the number of job titles and levels may exceed two dozen. Included are an attending physician, a resident from medicine, a chief resident from medicine, a consulting resident from surgery, a laboratory technician, a nurse supervisor, a staff nurse, an orderly, aides, volunteers, housekeepers and their supervisors, ward clerks, food services personnel and their supervisors, maintenance staff from the engineering department, respiratory therapists, etc. A housekeeping supervisor is responsible for all the housekeepers, a food service director is responsible for the range of food service activities in the institution, and the Director of Nursing is responsible for everything from the nursery to the operating room. Conflict is almost inevitable in trying to coordinate the activities of all these people in the best interest of the patients on the floor.

In the typical hierarchical organization, a problem, complaint, or change requires sending messages up the various chains of command and then having the middle managers—either the department heads or assistant administrators— coordinate their efforts, resolve the issue, and communicate the decision down their various command chains. The amount of communication involved in all of that carries a tremendous potential for distortion or incorrect interpretation. The matrix organization delegates large areas of responsibility and authority to an administrator on the unit, perhaps a nurse or manager. The people on the unit are initially responsible to this administrator, who coordinates all disparate areas. The major criticism of this approach is that, instead of one "boss," there are now two or three.

CENTRAL CONCEPTS

The traditional issues considered in discussions of structure are span of control, division of labor, departmentalization, and delegation.

Span of Control

Span of control is perhaps the most academic of all these issues, since there is no clearly right answer. The basic question here is, How many persons can a given manager effectively manage? The answer depends on the skill of the manager, the intensity with which he or she wants to manage, the quality of subordinates, the quality of the operating systems, and countless other factors. The condition of the physical plant may even have an impact on the issue of span of control. For example, if the health facility has a plant that is in excellent repair and does not need any major renovations or expansions, a manager will not have to hassle with the myriad problems of a poor plant and frustrated maintenance staff, and will be freed to deal with other people or problems.

Discussions of span of control usually concern an industrial organization. In those instances, it is relatively easy to identify the number of contacts managers are likely to have outside of their line position. In health care organizations, the problems of managing a staff are compounded by the problems of managing a medical staff and a host of regulatory agencies. It should be clear to any health care manager that, regardless of what the organization chart states, it is the rare physician who walks into the manager's office with the idea of seeing the "boss." The fundamental issue in health care organizational structure is that a major component of the organization, the medical staff, is effectively off the chart. Span of control, then, is a useful concept for certain portions of the administrative organization of most health care programs, but it is an unrealistic concept for many professional activities.

Division of Labor

The second central concept in organizational structure is division of labor. Jobs are organized in such a way as to divide specific functions appropriately. The prime motivating force behind the division of labor into the most appropriate and manageable tasks should be logic. In industrial organizations, logic plays an important role; however, in the health care field, logic is somewhat constrained by licensure requirements, power relationships, and tradition. In nursing, for example, the registered nurse (RN) has the authority to administer certain medications under the physician's orders, while the licensed practical nurse (LPN) works under more restrictions. Years of experience, maturity, and skill will never allow the LPN to function as an RN. At the next step up the ladder, on pain of dismissal or even worse, the RN cannot order a medication, stop a medication, or change it. Obviously, there are standing orders and various ways around this situation, but the fact remains that even a person who has developed the skill and experience to function in a higher role will not be able to function formally in this role. Despite their skill and knowledge, nurse-midwives are never granted a franchise similar to that which the least experienced general practitioner has for the delivery of obstetrical services, and there is no way the administrator of a hospital in which she works under the direction of the medical staff can restructure the clinical services so that she can function exactly as an obstetrician. So, in the health field the division of labor in many critical areas is more a function of tradition and licensure requirements than the logic of the system.

At a theoretical level, industrial engineers could come into the health care organizations, stopwatches in hand, and develop various schemes for maximizing the effectiveness and efficiency of the institution while minimizing the expenses. Their findings would likely involve reconstituting jobs and reorganizing relationships. The legal and social structure provides too many constraints about what could be reconstituted and thus reorganized, however.

In the best of all possible organizational worlds, a health care organization would be started from scratch; jobs would be defined, people who met the specifications for the jobs would be hired, and the organization would be set up in a functional way to meet relatively clear goals. In the health care field, as noted in an earlier chapter, goals are a bit diffuse. When compounded by the constraints of labor division, this diffuseness presents problems in establishing theoretical departments. At this point, it is interesting to consider how frequently both private industry and government reorganize and reconstitute their various departments. In the late 1970s Sears, Roebuck and Co. started emphasizing the importance of sales over profits, and the result was a massive selling effort by the various stores. A decline in profits resulted, since much discounting was taking place to spur sales. Each time Sears changed goals, a reorganization and rebalancing of the organization was required. Observers of both the federal and state health establishments will probably agree that these organizations have made reorganization their regular mode of operation.

Departmentalization

The third structural issue, departmentalization, takes place along traditional educational lines and, to a lesser extent, on professional functional lines. It should also be noted that some departmentalization takes place on purely political lines or, in some cases, economic lines. For example, one hospital studied had both a laboratory and a pathology department. These two departments in many respects had duplicate equipment and personnel, resulting in excessive laboratory and pathology costs for the patients. They were organized in this way primarily because of personality conflicts between the laboratory director and the pathologist. Further exacerbating the problem was the administration's interest in keeping tight control of the income in the laboratory, which was considered easier if the pathologist was not involved. From a general managerial perspective, the arrangement was senseless, but in terms of the politics of that organization it was necessary.

Delegation

A fourth area for consideration is that of delegation, passing the authority and responsibility for a given operation to those at different levels of the organization's structure. The classic concept is that responsibility and authority should function in concert. An individual who has the responsibility for carrying out a job should also have the authority to finish the job. In the automobile production factory, this might be possible, but in the health setting with its myriad subspecialists, the situation is more complex. A respiratory therapist might be sent down to see a patient who is having difficulty breathing. At what stage in the patient's distress is the therapist in charge, or the nurse, or the physician (which physician—the patient's family practitioner, surgeon, anesthesiologist, or psychiatrist)?

In general, health care organizations, most notably hospitals, manifest considerable confusion when it comes to organizational structure. Typically, they are organized along the axis of disease, age of patient, ambulatory status of patient, type of patient, and nature of supportive services. Hospitals usually have the following services: medicine, surgery, obstetrics, gynecology, and pediatrics. In more avant garde institutions, there is an ambulatory care service, which crosses all clinical barriers for the walking patient; an emergency service for the patient needing immediate care; and countless supporting services, ranging from the laboratory and x-ray to the laundry and cafeteria.

To say that the typical hospital organization chart is a hodgepodge is an understatement. It is a complete mess—full of dotted lines and direct lines of authority and responsibility that are meaningless. Who, for example, is responsible for the quality of professional care rendered by the respiratory therapist? The answer is simple: the head of respiratory therapy who, in turn, is responsible to a higher level of management, and eventually responsibility is traced up to the chief executive officer. The same chain can be followed to find who is responsible for the quality of lunch in the cafeteria. Now, who is responsible for the quality of surgical services delivered by Dr. Smith, a private practitioner who operates in the Jones Hospital seven times per week? The answers, despite all the organization charts, dotted and straight lines, become very fuzzy. It boils down to the fact that, for the most part, no one directs Smith; he is primarily responsible to himself. He certainly does not take orders from the elected chief of his service or the chief executive officer of the institution. He may negotiate with them, but views these as negotiations among equals.

The problem here, as with most other health care organizations, is that the organization's primary reason for being is not even on the organization chart (Exhibits 9-1 and 9-2). As an airline cannot function without pilots, a health care organization cannot function without physicians. While the airline does not have direct control over the minute-to-minute functioning of a pilot, there is no question in the pilots' mind that they work for the airline and that the airline has the authority and responsibility to schedule their activities, increase them (within limits), or change them—that is, the airline has purchased their skill and time and can use them to meet its objectives. Of course, pilots have the right to refuse and attempt to sell their skill and time to another bidder.

For the most part, the voluntary hospital functions on stand-by, awaiting the utilization of its services by a theoretically undependable physician. Undependable means that physicians schedule their day, week, month, year, or professional career to meet their own needs, not the needs of the institution. How many physicians, for example, would be willing to reschedule their vacations and/or operating schedules in order to accommodate the low census problems of the local hospital? It is difficult for the institution, of course, to plan rationally when it cannot directly control its major component or, conversely, to develop extraorganization chart mechanisms that allow it indirect control over this component.

Other health care organizations, such as group practices or government hospitals, function differently, not because they are organized differently per se but rather because the nature of the physician involvement is different. Typically, physicians do not simply join a fee-for-service multispecialty group practice but are invited to join on the basis of what they are likely to contribute economically and professionally to the practice. No physician can free-float into the organization simply by moving into the area. Second, expectations in terms of production are set either directly or indirectly for each new physician. In most cases, their

Exhibit 9-1 Organization Chart of 1,000-Bed Teaching Hospital

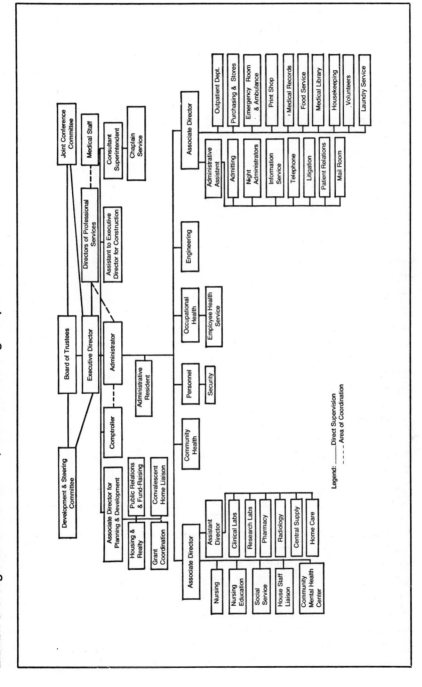

Exhibit 9-2 Organization Chart of 300-Bed Community Hospital

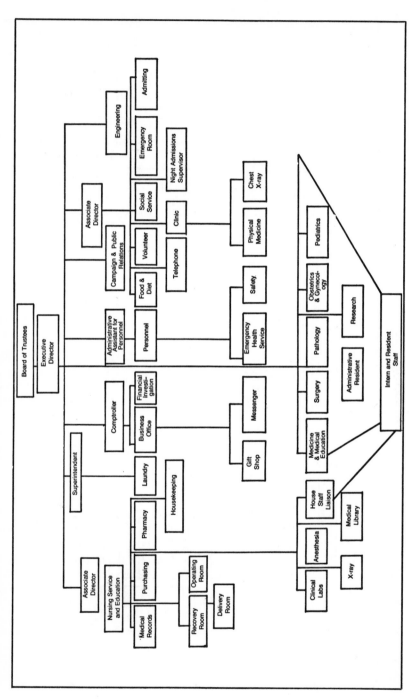

incomes are a direct function of their gross input into the practice. Third, support services are developed to help the practitioner practice more efficient and effective medicine. As the practice grows, the management of the support services may become so complex that a business manager is hired, and this manager may also take the responsibility for managing the time and expertise of the clinicians in their best financial and professional interests.

Two points about this private group practice should be made clear: first, the manager is an employee of the physicians; second, sometimes the manager has a better understanding of the physicians' best interests than they do. In all instances, however, the manager's authority and responsibility are derived from the group's members, and the manager is theoretically involved in negotiating with them, not ordering them. The skills needed by a negotiator are quite different from those needed by a person whose authority comes from a line position. Negotiators must act from a base of expertise and hard data, and they must have the ability to persuade and inspire loyalty for themselves and their ideas. Finally, they must deliver, lest a previous poor performance undermine their expertise the next time. Thus, for the manager in the group practice situation the "track record" is all important.

The most dramatic authority situation involves the physician in a naval hospital. Quite clearly, the person in charge is called the commanding officer. Until recently, all commanding officers at health care institutions were physicians, but in the past few years the Navy has allowed administrators to have command posts; however, the Navy has effectively restricted the authority of the nonphysician commanding officers by establishing the executive officer (next down in the chain of command) as the director of Clinical Services and making this officer responsible for all physician activities. De facto though, what authority does the commanding officer have? It depends on what authority the physician is willing to accept. Commanding officers prepare annual evaluations, and through this mechanism they can affect a career officer's chances for promotion or perhaps assignment. Within their own command, they can assign certain tasks and responsibilities, and they can use this power to reassign as a tool in negotiations. The authority to court-martial is for the most part irrelevant, since it borders on the absurd to court-martial a physician for behaving as an autonomous professional. Thus, even in a military organization, management must negotiate with professionals if performance is the objective. It may be concluded that, where the professional side of a health care organization is concerned, leadership and negotiation skills are far more important than formal structural position.

The nonprofessional components of the organization function according to the delineated structure in which authority and responsibility are delegated to various people, and approvals for action are required up and down the line. Negotiation and leadership skills are replaced with directives and technical expertise on the job.

Members of the staff in military hospitals are treated quite in accordance with their professional stature, which is also reflected in their rank. Although a physician could repeatedly arrive late in the morning and avoid discipline, the unfortunate corpsman who made a habit of such behavior could look forward to a meeting with the commanding officer. In effect, then, the organization functions both as a Theory X place and a Theory Y place—X for those on the organization chart and Y for those not on it.

As noted earlier, the value of structure is that it gives some indications about the members of the organization and their general responsibility and authority. It does not reveal very much about the quality of their relationships or how well they do their jobs. Structure is also, at least in part, clear. Theoretical assumptions can be made. Since process is harder to deal with than structure, and outcome is even more difficult to deal with, there is a tendency to believe that changes in structure will inevitably lead to changes in process and outcome. This point is illustrated not only by the seemingly continual changes at the Department of Health and Human Services, but also by the New York City Health and Hospitals Corporation. In the late 1950s and early 1960s, the solution to the problems of the municipal hospitals was considered to be the affiliation agreements between the voluntary and municipal hospitals. A later solution was the establishment of the quasi-independent Health and Hospitals Corporation. In 1979, the solution was the reestablishment of the Department of Hospitals as a municipal department and the decentralization of the total structure. As of yet, nothing has worked, despite the infusion of billions of dollars in salaries and the development of a massive organizational structure with a central office of hundreds of people.

VALUES OF ORGANIZATIONAL STRUCTURE

A clear value of a solid organizational structure is in the large multiunit organizations where it is imperative that response time be minimized. This organizational structure allows for policy development and policy interpretation, but precludes continuous communication between the top levels and the operating levels of an organization. The written policy is a critical communication tool that is interrelated to the organizational structure, since it is dependent on the authority of someone in the chain of command.

Any health care organization has at least two structures: one is written on a piece of paper and is an artistic representation of what people believe happens, and the second is a nonwritten structure that actually represents the authority and responsibility centers of the organization. Further, despite what any chart states, a significant component group of those responsible, not only for the well-being of the organization's constituents but for the well-being of the organization (perhaps its life) will not be on the chart.

A different and equally significant value of organizational structure is that the structure itself can be used as a medium for transmitting messages both inside and outside the organization. It is a means of emphasizing (or deemphasizing) functions and people, and it is also a way of establishing a person's authority over the organization and its events. For example, rarely does a senior level executive or a new president come into an organization without an almost ceremonial reorganization. By reorganizing, a person is flexing organizational muscle—in reality, little may have changed, but the message has been sent that a new person is in charge.

A new structure has also become the mechanism for announcing a realignment of power or function in the organization. In hospitals people may be moved from a department head status to an assistant or full vice presidential status. There is a difference between being the director of Planning, responsible to the vice president of Operations, and being the vice president of Planning, reporting to the executive vice president or the president. Restructuring is often a way of demoting someone without the actual embarrassment of moving that person a notch down—everyone is moved up, but that person remains in the same place or is shifted laterally.

In sum, organizational structure has its special values to any organization. However, structure is not static; it is clearly one of many important tools a manager has to utilize in the quest for desired outcomes. Integral with the notions of organizational structure are those of staffing. In a theoretical way, an organization is built on the basis of goals, objectives, and concepts of outcomes. Managers are usually taught not to build their structure around people. People, some writers urge, should be viewed as interchangeable. People are not interchangeable, however, particularly those valuable people who for whatever reason act as catalysts for the development and maintenance of an effective organization. Indeed, to satisfy these people, it is sometimes imperative that an organization be restructured to recognize their particular talents.

STAFFING

Staffing is perhaps the most critical function for which management is responsible. Through the kind and quality of staff recruited, management can exert its greatest influence on the organization. Staffing includes several distinct phases:

- the identification of an organization's short-term and long-term manpower needs

- the definition of the jobs that are likely to be required

- the development of specifications for persons who will be suitable for these positions

- the recruitment of staff

- the development of staff

- the evaluation of staff

An organizational structure question that must be resolved immediately is whether staffing functions shall be centralized or decentralized. A centralized model usually results in a personnel department, most often viewed as a supportive service to the entire organization. In this model, the personnel department might coordinate all requests for personnel, in effect acting as a clearinghouse and, to some extent, as an adjunct of the chief executive. For example, in a large teaching hospital in New York the chief executive was trying to cut operating expenses. One of his strategies was to have personnel slow down their entire staffing processes. Whereas in the past it might have taken four weeks to fill a vacant position, it now took twice that length of time. In view of the annual turnover at that institution, millions of dollars could be saved by this strategy.

In a totally decentralized model, all staffing decisions are made at lower possible organizational levels. In the hospital, for example, the outpatient pediatric clinic might theoretically have the authority and responsibility for developing its own staffing patterns and then implementing them. The problem, of course, is that staff cost money. Despite the apparent needs of a unit, the funds may not be available to support the staff. In some instances, funds from a money-rich program are used to support a deficit operation—but this is likely only when there is a centralized system or a high level of understanding about the need for the various components to support the total system. Certain departments in a university are clear money makers, while others are money losers. Rare is the law or business school that does not generate considerably more revenue than it expends. On the other hand, the art and history departments are usually at the deficit end of the budget. For the university to be a total university, however, all the elements are necessary, and the fiscally strong must in fact subsidize the fiscally weak.

In the reality of health care organizations, there is a mixed centralized/ decentralized model of authority and responsibility for staffing, despite the fact that most organization charts suggest that the structure is totally centralized. Typically, the planning for manpower needs goes on at a rather low organizational level, such as a program or department. Depending on the power of that unit— power being a function of its fiscal strength potential and its importance to the organization and/or the personalities involved—the plan will either be implemented by the central functionaries (for example, personnel) at the direction of the unit, or it will be implemented by the unit itself. The structure itself does not dictate how the decision process will flow, but the uncharted power relationships dictate the course of action.

The value of the decentralized approach is that the process can be streamlined and the response time to meet the needs of a unit can be minimized. On the other hand, decentralization precludes comprehensive staff planning and may result in higher costs because of problems, such as when a given program recruits a person at a salary that is out of line with those in other units. A centralized system provides broad guidelines within which each unit makes its own decisions. In certain industrial situations in which operating divisions might be competing with each other, such staff decentralization would appear to be more sensible; however, in health care organizations, where careful articulation is almost mandatory, decentralization would appear to be a weaker approach.

Identification of Manpower Needs

In practice, a health care institution can either develop an organized and systematic method of evaluating its physician manpower needs, or it can hope, pray, and muddle through. Unfortunately, most health care organizations choose the latter mode, which generally means that the decision to hire a new staff member can originate from any one of several places in the organization and for a variety of reasons. In one hospital, for example, the administration added a physician to the ambulatory care group because he was a prestigious medical staff member who was interested in scaling down his practice and the hospital wished to retain his patients. A "problem of success" arose, however. The established physician brought to the ambulatory care group enough patients for his scaled-down practice, plus patients for the other group members. Indeed, shortly after he joined the ambulatory care group, another physician had to be added to handle the increased volume of business. Thus, the addition of one new person actually created the need for a second. However, the question as to whether the size of the group or the scope of its services reflected the needs of the community had never been addressed.

In another case, a group of physicians decided to add a full-time physician to the staff because they "felt" that there was a two-week to three-week wait for nonemergency treatment and that such a delay was excessive. The new person did not fill a need, and several months after he arrived it was necessary for him to be discharged. What had occurred? First, the "clinical impression" of the two-week to three-week wait, based on only a few shreds of evidence, was incorrect. Indeed, some persons waited that long to be admitted, but it was usually to accommodate their own schedule and not the physician's. Also, a demand for increased service was peaking in that community—something that analysis of past usage patterns would have disclosed and that demographic analysis could have explained.

Definition of Jobs

Both systems require a beginning point and that is the definition of the job to be performed. This then returns to the theoretical notions of structure. It is necessary to know exactly what jobs are required and, further, what specifically persons working in those jobs are going to do. The kind of physicians needed to develop a group practice depends on what the practice has as its objective. If they want to be a primary care group practice, they want physicians who will provide first contact routine medical care to patients of all ages. Excluded from the practice will be surgery other than the most minor types and long-term psychiatric care. The job description, then, explains the nature of the job and provides a general outline of the organization's expectation. It should also answer some fundamental questions: What are the duties to be performed in the job? How does this position relate to other positions in the organization? Who supervises the physician? Whom does the physician supervise? Together this reveals what the authority and responsibility of this job are. Theoretically, an organizational crossword puzzle can be made of all the job descriptions; if fitted together, they would generally indicate what the organization is de facto about.

Job Specifications

The statement of the job specifications emanates from the job description and, although it has similar components, it actually provides a list of qualifications that a suitable candidate should possess. For example, a job specification statement might include such obvious requirements as a license to practice in the state, along with more discriminating factors such as board certification or specialty. (Some job specifications identify needed value orientations or behaviors.) In the earlier example, the kind of physician to be recruited obviously should be from one of the primary care specialties such as family practice, internal medicine, or pediatrics; a neurologist, dermatologist, or thoracic surgeon would be inappropriate. While the process of preparing and updating job descriptions and translating those descriptions into specifications can be time-consuming, sometimes tortuous, it can lead to a firmer understanding of the position for which someone is being recruited and a sharper focus on the type of person needed to fill the position.

Recruitment

Perhaps the most critical function in staffing is recruitment. The objective of any recruitment effort is to hire the person best suited for a position. Every organization has its own specifications for a given job; in order to maximize its potential for finding the "one person who fits," it is suggested that the organization attempt as broad a search as possible. This strategy is not universally accepted, however. Some believe that a narrower and more discreet recruitment effort has a higher payoff both in terms of finding people and in terms of building the organization's image. By letting as many people as possible know that a search is underway and that all replies will be confidential, one can often identify candidates who were believed to be unavailable.

The various methods of recruitment that should be considered are inhouse recruiting, colleague inquiries, employment agencies, professional journal advertising, and newspaper advertising. The more clearly the job is defined, including the conditions of employment, the better the quality of the responses. For example, if an advertisement for an associate administrator in Florida states that compensation is dependent on experience and education, a pool of candidates will apply, ranging from recent graduates to senior administrators who are looking toward a financially viable retirement. Therefore, perhaps the advertisement should be for an associate administrator with five to seven years experience; starting salary $38,000.

Inhouse Recruiting

The logical first step in any search process is inhouse recruiting. Basically, it is a review of the persons within the organization to ascertain whether one of them is qualified to fill the vacant slot. A second dimension of such a process is that it allows the administration to keep the communication lines with the staff open so that the recruitment process is not viewed as a threat and information about available candidates can be exchanged. In earlier chapters we illustrated the importance of this approach with the example of the innovative manager.

Colleague Inquiries

One of the most popular search methods is writing letters to friends in the field and other appropriate persons, such as university department chairmen and staff of major hospitals. Responses to these letters vary from no answer to a deluge that includes the resumés of entire groups. If truly handled on a personal basis, the letter-writing process is time-consuming and expensive. It also tends to place a burden of increased correspondence on the recruiter, who may have to respond to requests for additional information or explain why a friend's choice was not selected.

Employment Agencies

A third strategy is the use of professional recruiting services. Organizations that provide such services include certain public accounting firms, national management consulting firms, and a host of executive search firms. In general, these firms secure candidates through the use of some advertising, a great many personal contacts, and files that have been developed over the years. The major advantage of these services is that they can identify and screen candidates in a fairly quiet, indeed sometimes anonymous, way. The primary disadvantage is that many of these organizations have limited experience and understanding of the health field, thus limiting their ability to evaluate candidates properly. Another unrelated but significant problem is that their fees can run as high as 20 percent of a year's salary.

A variation on the agency theme is the recruitment that is done by such professional organizations as the American Group Practice Association or the Medical Group Management Association. Somewhat like registries, these organizations attempt to provide candidates to institutions in search of a staff.

Advertising

Advertisements in professional journals are a popular and relatively inexpensive way of developing a candidate pool. Basically, there are two types of journals that can be used—the classic professional journal, such as *Hospitals* or the *New England Journal of Medicine,* or the various controlled circulation journals. Although the cost of such advertisements is low and the readership is high, time lag is a problem. For example, there are cases where jobs are filled by candidates attracted via other media before the journal advertisement appears.

An alternative that is becoming increasingly popular is specialized newspaper advertising—in particular, the health care opportunities section of *The Sunday New York Times.* Although these advertisements are not inexpensive, the response generally is quite good.

Basic Strategy

Persons considering a recruitment effort for professional level staff—major or minor—might want to consider the following, somewhat eclectic six-point strategy:

1. A mechanism for continuous assessment of the professional manpower needs of the organization should be developed—this could be centralized in personnel or decentralized in units with information provided to administration.
2. When a senior level or critical vacancy is projected, a small search committee of three to five persons should be established for the purpose of reviewing or developing the job description and specifications. Basic questions to be considered are whether the job is still needed and where the position should be located in the organization.
3. After the job description and specifications are finalized, the search committee should engage an outside consultant for one day or a half day as a reviewer.
4. A staff recruitment coordinator should place advertisements and send letters in order to develop a pool of qualified candidates.
5. Initial review of applicants should be done either by the search committee or in the case of technical positions perhaps a consultant. When the final group of candidates is selected, the search committee should interview and select.

6. After the selection has been made, the search committee and recruitment coordinator should evaluate the process and report on its effectiveness.

This six-point strategy is a general framework for thought. Recruitment is a time-consuming and expensive process that must be approached soberly and deliberately as recruitment mistakes are costly.

Those involved in the search should feel that their recommendations are being taken seriously. If the recommendations of people who have spent a good deal of time recruiting a new staff member are simply bypassed, this not only will be personally debilitating but will have a negative ripple effect throughout the organization. Universities are frequently guilty of such behavior. With much fanfare, a search committee is appointed to find a person to fill a high position; many busy persons are tied up for days or weeks; and, finally, the administration selects the person it wanted in the first instance. The appointment of a search committee has accomplished several things. First, it has bought the administration valuable time to make or negotiate its decision; second, it has provided the necessary image of democratic process to assuage a sometimes hostile faculty and a busy "equal opportunity" officer; and, occasionally, the committee identifies someone who might be appropriate to fill the job in question or some other job in the organization. Participation in the search committee ritual is a pastime some enjoy and others dislike intensely. In all cases, however, participants should feel that their time is not being wasted and that their efforts result in significant organizational contributions.

EVALUATION

Evaluation of structure or staffing assumes three key elements: (1) clear organizational goals, (2) identified production standards, and (3) objectivity on the part of those who are doing the evaluation and those being evaluated. Evaluation then is the art and science of organizational navigation—it is determining the organization's position in its chosen program area while simultaneously determining its efficiency and effectiveness. This is a rather tall order for the labor-intensive health care industry in which position, efficiency, and effectiveness are more likely to depend on the quality of staffing than on the quality of structure.

Can an excellent quality structure be effectively negated by a poor quality staff or, conversely, can an excellent staff overcome the problems inherent in a poor structure? Countless examples can be cited where a structure looks impressive on paper, but the organization itself simply does not function because the members of the staff are simply inadequate. For example, a few years ago, a university-based health services research organization failed completely in spite of the fact that its organizational design was based on that of one of the most successful research and development consulting firms in the United States. The organizational design was even translated architecturally in a way that emphasized the equality of all staff and their functions. The research center on virtually any indicator was a total bust, however. Within four years of its inception, despite massive transfusions of foundation start-up capital, it was practically out of business. The research center had failed to generate any important research or funds for further operation. There was almost 100 percent staff turnover, and the quality of those coming in was considerably below that of those leaving. It was extremely difficult to attract researchers; overall morale was extremely low; and, finally, the research organization had lost its credibility on the campus, thus making it even more difficult to secure funds from the university.

Why had this happened when a previously successful structure had been utilized? The success of the structure in the previous organization was a result of the clarity of its purpose and the quality of its staff. Structure itself does not generate quality, but quality may require major changes in structure. In many senses, the focus on structure in this new health services research organization was an example of the leadership's overconcern with form and insufficient concern with substance. Greater care was apparently taken in developing the structure and the conceptual mechanism for making the structure work, such as who will meet with whom and when, than with more important issues, such as what kind of research the organization will do, how it will provide its funding, and how it will attract top quality researchers.

When this organization was analyzed, it often appeared that the top leadership considered high quality researchers unimportant, since the structure was expected to generate better work because of the equality and cooperation required among junior level people. The leadership was in no way malicious but, rather, naive. Although the leaders themselves were researchers, they apparently either understood little about how organizations functioned or were committed to concepts that simply could not function within a university environment. So there were two fatal flaws: a naiveness about goals and objectives, and a dogmatic commitment to a structure. The two flaws eventually brought the organization its problems: staffing.

Virtually everyone hired during the years of inception was expected, at least at the beginning, to express a belief in the organizational structure. Not to believe in the structure with its countless meetings and, to an extent, intellectual insults was to be deemed an inappropriate candidate for a job. Sometimes, a genuine commitment to the structure soured after a while, and the person either left or became one of the mutterers. The top leaders, committed to the structure in an almost religious way, were unwilling to explore its cost/benefit ratio and thus provided themselves with a staff that was unable to meet the goals that the university had for it—financial self-sufficiency and quality professional publications.

Perhaps one of the more absurd examples of how this structure wasted the time and energy of the staff was an all-day meeting that was billed as an attempt to solve some of the research center's problems. All the staff had been invited, since the structure dictated organizational equality despite financial inequality. The meeting was proceeding in a rather serious manner with several physician researchers venting their frustration with the way things had been progressing. One particularly promising person had just finished a rather emotional comment on his frustration with the center, his own inability to translate his energy into publications, and its implications for his future at the university. The leader responded by saying that he understood the points and needed time to think about them. Then, with the same seriousness of purpose, the leader asked a young staff member, a recent high-school graduate who ran the mimeograph machine, for his evaluation of the center. The young man replied that he felt the major problem was that lunch hours were scheduled at a bad time, since they did not coincide with those of his friends. In almost the same tone he had used earlier, the leader answered that he understood the seriousness of the point and needed time to think about it. The young researcher and some of his professional colleagues left the meeting at the next break and shortly thereafter resigned from the center. They considered the response to their problems within that structure inappropriate, and they believed the leadership was more concerned with the maintenance of the structure than their own and hence the organization's development.

An evaluation of either staff or an organizational structure must begin with the identification of goals or objectives. Then standards for performance can be developed, and measurements can be made to determine how well the standard is being met. For example, the standard for a private airline is probably making a profit. What then is the standard for the organizational structure? Probably, maximizing profit. Maximizing profit then can be translated into planes, pilots, routes, and schedules. The greatest planes in the world flown by the finest pilots are hardly important if an airline has poor routes and schedules. How many people are interested in flying on a 747 between Crowley, Louisiana, and El Paso, Texas? Assuming that the airline has good routes and schedules, it must get the aircraft to fly in an efficient manner and get passengers to fly on their aircraft. Is it worth the $50,000 plus to get a top flight captain to man the controls of a multi-million dollar 747? Considering the risk involved in the alternatives, not only is it worth the direct outlay for the salary and supporting staff, but it is also worth the continual investment in this person to ensure quality.

Health care organizations could learn some lessons from the airline industry. First, goals and objectives that are realistic and environmentally acceptable must be established. These goals are then translated into statements regarding the kind of people needed. Theoretically, these statements are turned into job descriptions and specifications, and then someone who can be evaluated on the basis of the job description and contributions toward the organization's goals is hired.

To some extent, the acceptable or likely workload is unknown for some people, and this can cause an organizational structure to change. On one occasion, for example, shortly after I had accepted administrative responsibility for a medical records department, I began to receive complaints about the slow turn-around time for patient summaries and the difficulty of getting records transcribed. After some investigation, it became apparent that a centralized transcribing system for medical records was needed. During this investigation, inquiries about acceptable work-load standards for medical record transcribers showed that, despite what appeared to be effective supervision, production had within it a range of 100 percent. Even the top producer was generating about 35 percent less than the norm for this job. Yet everyone looked busy; in fact, in the past few years, the supervisor had been given bonuses for her excellent supervision. Evidence now revealed, however, that this department was at least twice as big as it should have been and costing twice as much. With the new system, the department was restructured, and new standards became the basis for evaluation.

In some organizations, standards are so explicit that the standards themselves are part of the staffing process. For example, in one major university faculty, candidates are told during their interviews how many publications in which journals are necessary for contract renewal, promotion, or tenure. While at first glance that may seem rather arbitrary, it does set some rather clear expectations for the person considering the position. Further, it provides the standards for evaluation. There are many evaluation mechanisms and a great deal of literature on personnel evaluation, but the key to all of them is having a clear understanding of what is expected of the incumbent and how that person fits into the total organizational picture.

Eventually, each person who evaluates others is forced to rely on personal judgment; but to the extent that the evaluator understands what the organization is all about and has empirical evidence on a given person, judgment can be refined and made most equitable.

In sum, then, organizational structures exist to facilitate decision making and to provide a road map to an organization. The structure itself should not be the goal, however, but rather a means for people within the organization to operate in an efficient and effective manner. The organizational structure may have to be redesigned, based on how well (or poorly) these people do their jobs.

CASE STUDY

The Green Memorial Hospital Case

Located in an area approximately 40 miles north of New York City, the Green Memorial Hospital is a 207-bed acute care institution that offers a relatively complete range of inpatient services. It has a total active medical staff of 135, and most of them view Green as their primary affiliation. There are no full-time physicians employed at the hospital; however, there is one group of four radiologists who have been associated with the hospital for over 20 years, a group of anesthesiologists with equally long involvement at Green Memorial, and a pathologist who has spent his entire postresidency career of 13 years at the hospital.

Four years ago, the hospital entered into a contract with a group of physicians for the provision of emergency care. Patients who come to the emergency room are now seen by a member of this group (one physician is always on duty) and then referred to the on-call physician for follow-up. Ambulatory care is limited to physical therapy and some health education programs.

The hospital's board chairman describes it as an excellent quality community hospital. There is no interest on the part of the board, administration, or the medical staff in the hospital being a teaching institution or a tertiary care center for its region.

The present hospital director has been with the institution for 23 years. When he first came, the hospital had 141 beds, and he and an assistant administrator "ran" the hospital. By 1970, the hospital had expanded to its present size and a second assistant was hired. The organization chart then was as shown in Figure 9-1.

Figure 9-1 Organization of Green Memorial Hospital in 1970

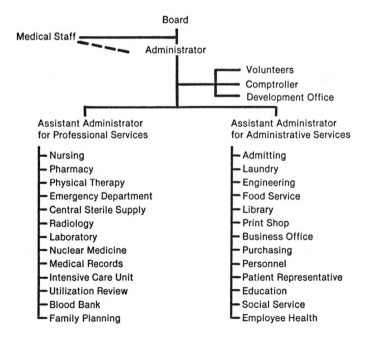

Figure 9-2 Proposed Organization of Green Memorial Hospital in 1980

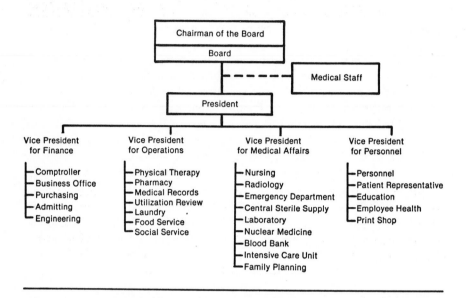

In 1980, the director announced his retirement as soon as a new director could be found, and the board both began a national search for a new director and engaged a consultant to review the organizational structure. The consultant's basic recommendation was to reorganize under a corporate form; toward that end, he offered the organization chart shown in Figure 9-2.

Discussion Questions

1. What are significant differences between the first and second chart?
2. What is implied in this new structure in terms of power relationships?

Chapter 10

Financial Management of Health Care Organizations

Many managers in health care institutions have only limited training or education in the field of financial management. However, they need a basic understanding of four major topics: (1) the financial organizations of health care institutions and programs, (2) the elements of health finance, (3) special issues in health finance, and (4) the budgeting process.

FINANCIAL COMPONENTS OF HEALTH CARE INSTITUTIONS

Most managers are involved with health care organizations in which the ultimate authority for financial decisions is in the hands of a board, which is required by corporate charter. This top level of financial management may or may not actually be involved in the financial management of the organization, depending on the power of the board. If it is indeed powerful, then that power more likely than not will be exercised through the purse strings. If it is not powerful, then it may simply act as a rubber stamp, or it may not be involved in the financial decisions at all. Quite often, boards take a middle-of-the-road position and act on annual budgets, any capital expenditure over a certain amount of money, or any major change in program that affects or risks the financial health of the organization.

Within larger organizations and/or larger boards, the functions related to finance may be delegated to a finance committee. This committee may have limited direct authority, or it may simply be a fact-finding group for the entire board. There is, of course, no simple formula for how all this should work. The key point is that, in many organizations, the board is ultimately responsible and does indeed exercise that responsibility.

It should be noted that the board is under no obligation to select only "financial wizards" to serve on the finance committee or to be their guiding light on financial

157

matters. In some instances, a board's finance committee is composed of lawyers or businessmen who have no particular expertise in finance, much less health care finance, and have learned what they need to know by experience through the years. For example, in one hospital, the long-time board treasurer was the owner of a small business who had no knowledge of the intricacies of health care finance. On one hand, such a situation is helpful in that the staff must make its case understandable to those who have only a general understanding of finance. On the other hand, in such a situation, the board is almost entirely dependent on staff for its information and then is, in a sense, captive of its own employees.

Within the health care organization or program, the focus of financial activities is the comptroller, vice president for finance, or treasurer—the nomenclature is so unstandardized that the same position may have scores of different titles. Most of these people are trained in accounting; sometimes they are certified public accountants, and occasionally they have special training in finance. Regardless of title, these people are the chief financial officers of their respective organizations and play a major part in developing and policing the systems that gather, analyze, and interpret financial and related operational data. In some organizations, this person and his or her staff play a key role in all managerial decisions, since they most often have the clearest understanding of the financial implications of any decision.

The major problem with such an accounting and finance staff (and some might say their major value) is that they often lack experience and perspective on health care operations. For example, most of the training programs in accounting and finance focus on the for-profit sector of the economy; entering the not-for-profit sector with its slightly different systems, new nomenclature, and different objectives presents problems to a person trained with a different value system and tools that are only useful when modified. To make up for the deficiencies, many organizations send promising individuals to special training programs and encourage them to enroll in the various health-related professional societies. Such educational and professional involvement serves two major purposes: it acquaints these people with the nature of health care organizations and their concerns, and it assists them in utilizing their professional skills to maximum effectiveness in the organization.

Other sources of manpower for this group of staff are the large public accounting firms. Until recently, the "Big 8" firms were primarily involved in the auditing side of health care; however, they have now expanded their areas of interest and expertise by becoming involved in financial feasibility studies and a range of management consultant activities. It appears that they are an excellent training ground for potential accounting and finance staff for health care organizations. Because the tight pyramidal structure of these accounting firms causes them to jettison the majority of their junior staff, these firms are a source of experienced and well-trained personnel.

The administrator, whether the president or executive director, is the person who is held most closely accountable for the financial management of the organization. Usually, administrators are not formally trained in finance or accounting but rather are trained in general management, which no doubt has included some background in accounting and finance. Like most managers, however, administrators must depend on the accounting and finance specialists for financial input into decision making. In some ways, an administrator's lack of training in accounting and finance is an obvious limitation; on the other hand, the administrator's primary value is in having a broad perspective on the problems and opportunities for the institution. So, for example, one administrator pushed ahead on a money-losing geriatric program because she felt it was important to the long-range interests of the relationship between her hospital and community. From a purely financial perspective, it might have been a bad decision; from a totally political perspective, it was certainly a reasonable choice.

Others in health care organizations are important in the financial management of an organization. Among these people are business office staff, who are involved in the credit and collection systems of the organization; data processing people, who are involved in the systems that set up and record transactions; purchasing staff, whose decisions affect the cash flow and hence the financial health of the organization; the personnel department, which through its policies affects turnover, vacation substitutions, and a range of other activities that can be translated into dollars and cents.

Essentially then, any health care organization operates with a series of cash registers that, if properly utilized, take in (or ensure the receipt of) revenues and disburse money in an organized and objective-related way. The nurse on the patient care floor of a hospital must ensure that the proper form is filled out when the laboratory test is ordered; otherwise, the business office does not bill the patient for the service. If the patient is not billed, then the organization has expended resources, such as the nurses' and laboratory technician's time, the machinery and supplies to perform the test, and all the overhead systems necessary to support the laboratory, without even the opportunity to be reimbursed. Thus, everyone in an organization is part of the revenue-generating function.

ELEMENTS OF HEALTH CARE FINANCE

Taxes

Health care organizations that are incorporated as for-profit organizations or are partnerships are taxed as any other organization is taxed. Most hospitals and a number of other institutions and programs, however, are incorporated as not-for-profit organizations and, therefore, are exempt from a range of federal, state, and local taxes under Section 501c3 of the Internal Revenue Code. This exemption does not preclude these organizations from making a profit or force them to operate at the break-even point, or even require them to lose money; rather, it requires that any profit made by such an organization must not directly benefit any single person or group of stockholders.

In general, the tax laws differentiate between related and unrelated income. Income from activities that are related to the operation and objectives of the organization, such as a profit-making cafeteria run by a large group practice for the convenience of the staff and patients, is tax-exempt. Clearly unrelated income would be taxable. For example, if a not-for-profit organization owned a spaghetti factory, the profits from the spaghetti factory would be taxable before they could be transferred to the not-for-profit organization. Farfetched example? Not really, since the Mueller Spaghetti Company was owned by New York University's Law School. There is, as in most tax law, a gray area of questionably related income. There has been some litigation regarding physicians' office buildings. Is the profit generated by such a facility taxable or not? In the cases that have been considered so far, the rulings have tended to accept the hospitals' argument that having the physicians on the campus of the facility is in the best interests of the patient.

Philanthropy

Occasionally, a wealthy benefactor wills a hospital or university millions. While that type of philanthropy is becoming rare, philanthropy on a smaller scale has continued for the past several decades; however, as a percentage of total revenue, it has declined. Philanthropy is important to an organization for spiritual as well as financial reasons. Spiritually, it tells the organization that it has friends and supporters, and in today's often hostile climate of management and regulation, such statements of support are comforting. From a financial perspective, philanthropy provides funds; however, many of the philanthropic gifts that health care organizations receive are specially targeted funds, i.e., given for a single purpose, such as a building or a program endowment. When money is put into an endowment, the use of the principal is restricted, and the interest is available for the purposes of the endowment.

A few of the problems facing health care organizations in terms of philanthropy include the source of the money, the restrictions placed on the money, and the cost of getting the money. When money is given, it appears to be less often transferred to the recipient in an unrestricted fashion than it was in the past. The problem with conditions on the money is that operational costs are rarely endowed; thus, for example, money may be provided for a new classroom and laboratory building at a hospital or university, but not for maintenance, heat, or cleaning the facility—costs that are sometimes too high for an organization to bear.

Finally, it should be noted that it takes considerable time and money to raise funds for any organization. Health care organizations must compete for limited charitable dollars with a range of other social programs. Some institutions employ full-time or part-time fund-raisers, while others hire consultant fund-raisers.

Operating Finances

Revenues

Revenues to health care organizations can be broken down into two categories: operating and nonoperating. The operating revenues are generated by the clients or patients who request the services that the organization is in business to offer. The nonoperating income is that which is generated independent of the patients in the organization, although it is directly related to the organization's existence and mission.

Operating income from patients may be financed by one of a variety of sources, including the government through Medicare or Medicaid and insurers, such as Blue Cross, Blue Shield, or one of scores of other private carriers. Each of these different payers operates with a slightly different set of reimbursement rules for services, and this translates into different billing and often different collection services. The income itself is generated by the patient who uses a hospital room, operating room, ancillary services (pharmacy, laboratory, x-ray), or professional services. In hospitals, because of differing agreements with the various payers, patients with similar diagnoses and treatment regimens being treated by the same physician in similar accommodations may, in fact, generate different revenues for the hospital. This is analogous to an airplane; despite the fact that all the passengers are flying between the same two cities, they are not all paying the same fare. Some are paying first class fare; others are paying full tourist fare; others are paying a 14- to 21-day fare; others are paying a 45-day excursion fare; others are traveling on half-fare coupons; others, on tour-based fare, and so forth.

Nonoperating revenue comes from grants for projects or development, philanthropy, and other activities, such as parking lots, cafeterias, and gift shops. This income is important, particularly when operating revenues are tight, since funds generated from these sources can often provide the seed money for future development and thus help the organization maintain a competitive edge in its area.

Expenses

The other side of the financial equation is expenses. In most health care organizations the major expense is clearly salaries. Depending on the organization, anywhere between 40 percent and 70 percent of the expenditures will be in salaries. Other expenses include cost of supplies, light, heat, malpractice insurance, bad debt allowances, maintenance of the physical facility, and so forth.

Capital Financing

The acquisition of money for capital projects, i.e., for major expenditures that relate to purchasing, restoring, or expanding buildings, property, and major pieces of equipment, is a problem for a health care organization. In the past few years, sources of capital financing have been primarily philanthropy (10 percent), taxable bonds (9 percent), retained earnings (13 percent), and tax-exempt securities (36 percent). In the not too distant past, the government, through its Hill-Burton and related programs, was a major source of capital financing to the hospital segment of the health industry. Indeed, many hospitals owe their very existence to the Hill-Burton program.

Taxable bonds are not the preferred route for capital financing because of the difficulty hospitals face in competing with private bonds and the high interest rate that they must offer in order to make their bonds marketable and attractive investments. Retained earnings are an attractive method, but it is hard for most health care organizations—particularly hospitals—to accumulate significant surpluses. Any surplus is usually fairly well wiped out by inflation, a new salary scale, or unanticipated expenditures, such as energy costs. Retained earnings are essentially the "profit" of the institution. Some argue that the depreciation costs passed on to patients through their insurers should, in fact, be placed aside for future capital expenditures and not be used for operating expenses.

The method of choice for most large health care organizations is the tax-exempt bond route, which allows the hospital to issue bonds either in its own name or through the auspices of a state bonding authority. Regardless, the interest rate offered to the potential investor is lower than that on a taxable bond because the interest from the bond is exempt from state and federal taxes. To qualify for the bond market, the institution must undergo a level of scrutiny that until recently was unusual in the health care field. This scrutiny involves a time-consuming and expensive financial and marketing feasibility study that basically examines the present and probable future financial health of the organization. Elements of the investigation include the present and probable future demand for services, the nature of the organization, its financial health as manifested by its operating statements (including balance sheets and statements of revenue and expenses), and its operating history. These data are usually assembled for a package that is offered as a prospectus for potential investors.

Lacking other sources of financing, an organization can simply turn to the private world of commercial and savings banks and attempt to obtain money from them. When money is available, however, the interest rates are likely to be the highest. It should also be noted that, depending on the projects being considered, different states have unique arrangements for getting money, such as state dormitory or educational facilities money, and the federal government sometimes lends money through various development authorities. Aggressive and creative organizations have found money in rather unusual places.

SPECIAL ISSUES

A variety of special issues and concerns face those involved in health care, particularly (but not limited to) those involved in hospital financing.

Cost of Regulation

One of the reactions to the barrage of new regulations that have hit the health field in the past decade has been criticism of the regulations themselves as the cause of (or at least a major contributor to) the problems to be solved by regulation. It is argued that regulations are developed to stem the sharp increase in hospital costs, but hospital spokesmen and politicians note that the regulations themselves are costly to implement and thus drive up hospital costs. Kinzer, in his book on regulation in the health care industry, states that a 471-bed hospital in Massachusetts would incur an additional $354,000 in annual expenses to meet the costs involved in complying with various regulations.[1]

Drake, an executive with the American Hospital Association, notes that, based on the general regulatory tone in this country, the "total direct incremental compliance cost of hospital regulation in 1978 [was] from $0.9 billion to $2.4 billion for short-term acute hospitals." He also states that if the New York State model of regulation were adopted nationwide, the costs would be closer to $6 billion.[2]

Acknowledging the cost of regulation, the 1980 Republican health plank included the following statements:

> Health care costs continue to rise, farther and faster than they should, and they threaten to spiral beyond the reach of many families. The causes are the Democratic Congress' inflationary spending and excessive and expensive regulations.

> The prescription for good health care is deregulation and an emphasis upon consumers' rights and patient choice.[3]

The cost of regulation can probably be categorized in three ways: recurring, capital, and investment. Recurring costs are those associated primarily with workers who must be employed to provide the documentation necessary for compliance with regulations. Capital costs are usually one-time expenditures to bring a facility up to certain standards, such as meeting life safety code requirements. Investment costs are those associated with developing certificates of need or any steps in the planning process that might precede a certificate-of-need application. For health care organizations, many of these costs are recoverable from third-party insurers, and do not present a significant internal management problem. However, there are other costs of regulation that are less clear, such as needed programs that were not launched or were delayed because of the regulatory process, but were finally developed at a higher price than originally anticipated.

In general, discussions of cost center around the new regulatory programs such as rate setting and certificates of need; one rarely finds cost-of-regulation discussions about the more established regulatory programs such as licensure or life safety codes. Debate on the cost issue will no doubt continue for many years; however, one should certainly balance this debate with a discussion of the benefits that will accrue to society as a result of regulation.

Biles, Schramm, and Atkinson suggest that rate setting is taking hold and demonstrating an ability to cut into the rapid rise of health care costs.[4] Perhaps a more important set of findings comes from a report on the Massachusetts Institute of Technology study of regulation, which notes, for example, that

> up to 60,000 lost workday accidents and 350 deaths were avoided in 1974 and 1975 due to OSHA rules on workplace safety . . .

> crib safety standards have reduced crib-related injuries to infants by 44 percent since 1974.[5]

The costs of health regulation as well as its benefits remain unclear and are likely to do so for the foreseeable future, both because the regulatory system is still developing and the costs are difficult to ascertain. Perhaps in the future the health industry will behave like the trucking and airline industries have with regard to regulation; after decades of regulation, they actively opposed deregulation that was proposed and implemented during the Carter administration. What they apparently had discovered was that the economic benefits of regulation outweighed the economic costs.

Cost Allocation

The trick for most health care organizations, in particular hospitals, is to maximize their revenue or reimbursements for the services they offer. As previously noted, patients, like airline passengers, each pay a different amount for the same service. Blue Cross, Medicare, and Medicaid each pay the "reasonable costs" of services—but each of these three payers defines "reasonable" differently. Commercial insurers, on the other hand, tend to pay charges, and private, self-paying patients are effectively in the worst category (for themselves, not the organization) because they pay posted charges that are essentially what the traffic will bear. Indeed, it should be noted that even among the scores of Blue Cross plans, there is considerable variation as to what is paid for and what is disallowed.

All of this being the case, it is in the best interests of the institution to allocate costs in such a way as to maximize reimbursement. For example, if inpatient costs are more generously reimbursed than outpatient costs, as much overhead as possible may be allocated to the inpatient units. Within the commonly accepted principles of accounting and finance, there is considerable discretion for cost allocation to maximize reimbursement. In some instances, institutions have reorganized to take advantage of the reimbursement formulas. Caution should be used, however, because reimbursement strategy is one of the most complex and technical problems facing health care organizations. For that reason, the expenditures involved in utilizing specialized consultants' services have often been worthwhile investments.

Cost Containment, Avoidance, and Reduction

Much of the regulatory activity that has occurred over the past few years in the health field has been intended to prevent further escalation in the costs of health care. In general, several strategies can be followed by organizations wishing to contain, avoid, and reduce costs. These strategies include paperwork improvements, productivity improvements, scheduling, and training.

Typical of the problems faced by many health care organizations are cash shortages, overstaffing, poor utilization of present staff, low productivity, and equipment breakdown. With regard to cash shortages, an organization can establish a budgeting system that contains mechanisms for more accurate forecasting. In order to ensure appropriate cash flow billing and collection, systems must be developed and maintained. The key word is systems. It is always amazing to find out how poorly many health care organizations handle billing. Even a day's delay in sending out bills or asking for reimbursement is costly to an organization.

Rare is the organization that does not have too many staff in certain departments and poorly utilized staff in others. Either situation is very costly and can be alleviated by better planning and coordination of personnel actions. It cannot be emphasized too strongly that, in a labor-intensive industry such as health care, it is imperative that all steps be taken to ensure the most efficient and effective utilization of staff. This, unfortunately, is not often done, and some institutions retain expensive anachronisms, such as doormen, that are really throwbacks to a bygone era not so much of amenities but of cheap labor.

The related problem of low productivity could be a function of numerous factors. For example, low productivity may result from recruiting inappropriate staff, i.e., people with poor skills or the wrong kind of skills. An emergency department that hires a recently retired psychiatrist from the state government system must expect a different level and type of productivity from this person than from a young physician who had just completed residency in family practice. Productivity problems, as noted in the earlier example involving medical records, are often the result of poorly developed expectations for workers—a problem that can be solved by analysis of the jobs in question and related activities. Sometimes low productivity is related neither to production standards nor to the caliber of staff but rather to the basic systems for getting the job completed. This can best be seen in any process that requires input or material from any other component of the organization before it can proceed with its work flow. On the Ford assembly line, each of the various functions must be carefully articulated with the previous ones, and materials must be readily available. Without the wheel assembly, the tires cannot be put on, and so forth. Even within health institutions there is a considerable amount of integration required: the operating room schedule can become bogged down because of a breakdown in central supply; the business office can be slowed down because information does not arrive from the ancillary service areas or other revenue-generating parts of a facility. Any of these breakdowns are expensive simply because they result in unproductive staff time that must be paid for.

Management of Working Capital

Working capital can be thought of as those assets of the organization that are essentially current, such as cash, accounts receivable, and inventory, as opposed to its fixed assets, which might include land and buildings. The basic idea of working capital management is to utilize the current assets to keep the organization in the strongest financial position. In considering this issue of management of working capital, there are three especially important areas of concern: inventory, accounts receivable, and accounts payable.

Inventory

The basic concern in inventory control is to balance the cost of not having enough with the cost of having too much. Inventory costs money to purchase, and this money is essentially out of circulation until the inventory is used and then converted back to cash. In addition, inventory costs money to store. A final problem is that some items have a limited life; if not used during their "shelf life," they must be destroyed. A typical question facing a health care manager is how many disposable syringes to buy: a day's supply at a time, a week's supply, a month's supply? It is not so very different from the question the consumer faces when the supermarket has a special on tuna fish. How many cans should the consumer buy? If the consumer uses all the money for tuna, then none is left over for other needs. A second limitation is space, and a third limitation is shelf life—should tuna that was bought five years ago be used? So it is with the disposable syringes—all the money in central supply cannot be allocated to this item, even if it is bargain-priced and the cost is going up in the future, since central supply needs other items that are equally important.

An additional factor in the inventory equation may be the likely availability of the product from suppliers. The reason most people do not carry large inventories of groceries is that large inventories are readily available in neighboring markets. Several years ago, a hospital in Brooklyn, New York, took this approach with its oxygen systems—since oxygen tank supplies were readily available, why should they go on a more expensive (capital-wise) central system that required them to have a large storage tank on their premises? Rather, they reasoned, it would be better to buy tanks in small amounts and bring in new supplies a few times weekly. This worked well until a strike occurred and the oxygen tanks could not be found. Finally, an imminent disaster was averted when oxygen was located some 50 miles away in New Jersey. When things settled down, the hospital began work on its new central oxygen system—the experience of the institution changed its attitudes toward the cost/benefit ratios.

Accounts Receivable

Accounts receivable are an integral component of cash management, since they are the monies owed the organization for services rendered. Most health care organizations operate on a noncash basis; patients or their insurance companies are billed for services, and these bills take some period of time to collect. On the other hand, the organization has obligations to pay those staff who have rendered the services that generate the bills. A nurse is not told that she will be paid as soon as Blue Shield pays Mrs. Smith's bill. Rather, the nurse and the rest of the staff are paid on a periodic basis, even though a good deal of receivables do not come in on such a regular basis.

The key in accounts receivable is to set up an efficient billing and collection system so that bills are sent expeditiously with all the proper information (this is particularly important when dealing with the third party reimbursers) and that follow-up takes place. One hospital in New York City got so far behind in its receivables that at one time it had over $28 million in receivables. Over time, receivables can deteriorate to such a point that it becomes progressively more difficult to collect on them, particularly from private pay patients. There are no easy solutions to the accounts receivable problems, but the significance of organized systems must be emphasized. Organizations should carefully evaluate what have in the past been unacceptable alternatives, such as use of credit cards or the development of time payment schemes for patients. Finally, it must be recognized that a dollar collected today is worth more than a dollar collected in two months, and therefore the investment in a good system has clear financial merits.

Accounts Payable

To some extent accounts payable are the other side of the equation. They are monies the organization is paying out for services and supplies that it has acquired or is planning to acquire. The major account payable for most health care organizations is the payroll. From the organization's financial perspective, it is best if they can pay over the longest stretch possible; for example, they have a monthly payment of staff. This means 12 processings a year, and the organization has considerably more cash on hand during the month than under a weekly system where 52 processings a year are required and, of course, are more costly.

In business, suppliers often offer incentives for rapid payment such as one percent off the bill if paid within ten days. In one hospital, the working capital was so poorly managed (some argued that it was actually good management) that the institution was months and months behind in its payments. In some instances, suppliers had cut off deliveries to the institution until old bills were cleared up, and thereafter they would supply the hospital only if cash were paid for the supplies. Again, the key is having an organized system for paying obligations—but this system must be integrated into the total working capital system, which is designed to ensure that money owed the organization is received as rapidly as possible and that funds are properly expended in inventory.

Inpatient versus Outpatient Revenue and Expenses

A special problem faced primarily by hospitals, one about which there is a great deal of confusion, concerns inpatient versus outpatient revenue and expenses. First, it should be remembered that outpatient departments are essentially a large teaching hospital phenomenon. Outside of these large teaching hospitals, which offer a wide range of clinics providing ambulatory care to a large number of patients, outpatient departments usually mean places to go for ancillary services, such as physical therapy or perhaps an x-ray.

The objective in most institutions is to maximize total revenue. Of late, the litany among hospital administrators has been that outpatient services are big money losers, but they are maintained because they are an important community service. The "ambulatory careniks" sing a different song: outpatient departments are only money losers because the hospital unfairly apportions the overhead expenses of the hospital to that area.

As can be expected, the truth—if there is a truth in this question—is somewhere in between. An outpatient department serves a vital function to the inpatient side of the hospital. It often generates upwards of 20 percent of the admissions and a significant amount of revenues for the ancillary services. When costs are allocated, one method is through the mechanism of the step-down formula, which allocates costs of nonrevenue-producing areas to the revenue-producing areas. Invariably, outpatient departments come out with a deficit, not so much because they are receiving an inappropriate allocation of the expense but because they are not receiving appropriate credit for the revenues that they generate directly or indirectly. Perhaps a step-up formula is needed for properly crediting the source of the revenues in a hospital. All of this is tied together by the fact that, to a large extent, the financial health and well-being of a hospital is very much related to its occupancy rate. This rate can be greatly affected by the activity in the outpatient area, including the emergency room, which is the entry to the inpatient services for so many patients. These areas then are to an important extent the loss leaders of the institution.

THE BUDGETARY PROCESS

A budget is essentially a statement of expected expenses and expected revenues over a certain period of time. Most organizations have some sort of budget and a process that arrives at that budget. Some organizations, such as hospitals, must meet requirements of the federal government and sometimes state governments for budgets of varying lengths. Indeed, some states, e.g., Connecticut, use the budget as a key regulatory device. Also, virtually every government-run or government-financed program is required at the least to prepare a budget at its outset.

In theory then, a budget is a financial timetable, a plan for the organization that has been translated into dollars and cents. A different way of viewing the budget is that it is fundamentally a political document that oftentimes involves a complicated bargaining process within the organization. Thus, forecasting, or in some cases educated guessing, becomes a key element in the entire budgeting process. Because of the political nature of budgeting and the control that management has when it makes decisions affecting department budgetary levels, the budget and the process can become very significant management tools.

For practical purposes, there are three general types of budgets many organizations use: cash, capital, and expense. The cash budget is concerned with cash receipts and disbursements; it is developed to ensure that the business of the organization proceeds at a smooth pace. The capital budget is concerned with capital acquisitions, such as buildings, land, or equipment. Finally, the major budget is the expense budget, which is essentially a statement of the planned operation for a subsequent period of time. The output—that is, the budgetary document—does not vary on the face of it from organization to organization, but the process to get to that document does vary. In the end though, a financial document is prepared; some might be program-based, while others itemize each expense individually (hence are called line items). Regardless, with minor effort each type can be translated into the other.

Traditional Budgetary Process

The typical budgetary process has four stages: (1) dissemination of instructions, (2) preparation of initial budget, (3) review and adjustment, and (4) appeal. Dissemination of instructions is exactly that. The instructions to be followed in the preparation of next year's budget are sent to those people who have been designated responsible for their section of the budget. This is in reality the beginning of management's political statement about the budget and its seriousness about the budget. The first question is, Who prepares the instructions? Is budget preparation by fiat from the management or finance department, or is the instruction rulemaking process itself open for question and negotiation? The instructions must also contain some parameters and forecasts—again, an opportunity for management to use its control. For example, in the instructions it might say, "Because of our tight fiscal situation, do not budget any new positions in your department or plan expense for consumable supplies at a level of 2.25 percent higher than last year." Effectively, management has sent a stark message to the department through the process itself.

Another way management makes an important statement about the budget is by its choice of staff to prepare the budget. In one large teaching hospital, the department secretaries were responsible for budget preparation, while in another it was the clinical chief of the service.

Having read through and digested the mechanics of the instructions, someone within the department is now ready to prepare the initial budget. Within a given component, the budgetary process may reflect the entire organization's approach or the management style of that department manager. For example, the department may have an open process where members of the department discuss their plans for the coming year and the money needed to translate those plans into action, or the manager may decide what should happen next year and plan accordingly. Sometimes there is no room in the budget for more than incremental financial plans for the future. Thus, ambulatory care, which had a budget of X dollars for A number of patients, may expect a plus ten percent next year based on the experiences of the past two years and may therefore request more money for supplies to meet this anticipated demand. Such a request is likely to be granted with no problem, but the request for the extra staff member to meet the extra demand may result in tough negotiation.

Negotiation takes place at the next stage, review and adjustment at the next higher organization level—perhaps the second level of management. Here requests are pruned and coordinated. Since the final budget must be adopted at the highest management level (in many organizations, the board level), it is in everyone's interest to make sure that the document, when finally presented, is as defensible as possible. A strong defense of requests is possible when the forecasts are good and the requests are reasonable. At this review level, it is important to see that each department has interpreted the forecasting data properly and is using assumptions similar to those of other departments. Also, it is an opportunity to ensure that there is no duplication.

The budget is then returned to the originating department. Depending on management's approach, a final appeal to top management is possible. If the department secretary has prepared the budget, there will be few appeals, since the secretary is not likely to be in a power position; also, by asking the secretary to prepare the budget, management has said that they really consider the process just an academic exercise. On the other hand, if the process is serious and has consumed much energy of "powerful" department level personnel, an appeal process to override the decision of the coordinating managerial level may be necessary. Here, the case for an increase or change is again made, and the budget may be adjusted.

It should be remembered that the budget may be reviewed by the board's finance committee before it goes to the full board. At every one of these stages of review and negotiation, questions are asked; if clarifications are not forthcoming, the budget may not be adopted.

Negotiation is the key to this type of process. In many senses, top management and lower levels are negotiating. They are to a degree in an adversary position; and, to the extent that each is operating at a high level of competence, the organization benefits by the challenge. For example, different groups may have different forecasts based on different interpretations of trends; it behooves the organization to analyze these interpretations before making a decision on the budget. In the closed and managerially dominant system, the opportunity for interaction and negotiation is limited and, this author believes, does not function in the best interests of the organization.

Even the timetable of the budgetary process is a statement of how serious and open management is about the process. Too short a timetable gives management total control of the process and the input data for decisions, while a reasonable timetable gives the individual departments the opportunity to analyze their own experiences and plans. Finally, it gives them opportunity to undertake negotiations in an atmosphere that is nonpressurized.

Zero-Based Budgeting

Thanks in large part to President Carter, virtually everyone has heard of zero-based budgeting. In the United States, zero-based budgeting became popular after Texas Instruments introduced it in their company. Basically, their notion was not to deal with the status quo of each year's budget as a springboard for the next year's budgeting cycle, but rather to rebuild the entire budget from the beginning and rejustify all expenses from the beginning.

The core of zero-based budgeting is the "decision package," which is a document prepared at the program or department level and states what the unit's objectives and plans are and what it will take for the unit to operate at different levels. In the Georgia State Government program, the following instructions are provided:

> Each decision package represents the fund requirement to support particular levels of the operations. The first package of a series of packages is developed at a minimum level of operations for the function. Additional levels of effort are Base level, Workload and new and improved . . . the minimum level is a level of effort, expressed in terms of service and cost, below which it is not feasible or possible to operate the function at all; . . . the workload decision package is developed only where funds are needed to meet increased workload at the functional level . . . the New or Improved Decision Package is developed for a requested improvement of an ongoing operation of the function or for a requested new operation in a function.[6]

The net result of this process is that units within an organization are forced to justify their own existence in writing. Management then has the task of sorting through thousands of these decision packages and setting priorities for the organization that can be translated into the acceptance or rejection of given packages.

In a recent review article on the subject, Suver and Brown found that only a limited number of organizations have adopted the technique, that the universal experience has been that the technique requires considerable modification, and that in some instances it was simply inappropriate.[7] Obviously, it generates a monumental amount of work for all levels of management and, to an extent, assumes that the system of budgeting in place is not satisfactory—which may not be the case. It, of course, does have an important value to an organization in that it requires an organized approach to the budgeting process and provides comparative data. Finally, because of the minimum package approach, it helps the organization see what its base commitments are and allows it to prepare a financial plan in case of disaster. Perhaps its greatest value is that it challenges everyday thinking and forces a justification where one is rarely requested.

CASE STUDY

The Blue Hospital-Based Group Practice

Three years ago, the Blue Hospital received a grant from a private foundation to develop a hospital-based group practice. The hospital is a 294-bed not-for-profit facility located in a major midwestern metropolitan area. Its community has three other hospitals of comparable size, and all these other institutions have teaching affiliations with the local medical school.

The foundation grant gave the hospital the opportunity to reorganize its ambulatory services into a two-section unit: the emergency service and the Blue primary care group practice. The original group had three family practitioners. Within a year of its opening, they added a full-time pediatrician and a full-time internist. It now appears that the group needs to expand again, but the anticipated addition of three physicians will require the physical expansion into space utilized by other departments—specifically, the cast room, the emergency department, and admitting. It is estimated that such an expansion will cost $97,714 and that the certificate-of-need process can be avoided.

To date, the present five group practice physicians account for 6.7 percent of the hospital's inpatient days. Additionally, they have been good for community relations, particularly during the first two years of their operation.

Prior to the group's establishment, key medical staff leaders were unhappy with the idea of a hospital-based group practice, since they viewed the then nonexistent group as a political and economic threat. The problems between the group and other medical staff have not materialized, and it now appears that one of the physicians formerly antagonistic to the group wishes to join it. Next year the foundation's subsidy to the group of $82,500 per year will be discontinued; if the subsidy were eliminated immediately, the group would be several thousand dollars shy of the break-even point. (See Table 10-1.)

Table 10-1 Financial and Activity Data on Blue Hospital Group Practice

Budget
　Revenues

Physicians	$398,780.00
X-ray	43,220.00
Laboratory	21,500.00
Other	9,500.00
Less write offs, discounts, etc.	10,000.00
Total operating revenue	$ 473,000.00

　Expenses

Administrative expenses	$ 27,500.00
Depreciation of building and equipment	44,000.00
Physician compensation	210,000.00
Staff compensation	97,000.00
Fringe benefits	62,000.00
Medical and surgical supplies	25,000.00
Office supplies/services	15,000.00
Professional insurance	21,000.00
Telephone	9,000.00
Consultants	10,000.00
Equipment leasing	5,000.00
Postage	5,000.00
Utilities	20,000.00
Miscellaneous	5,000.00
Total expenses	$ 555,500.00

Foundation grant $82,500.00

Patient Activity
Annual average of 325 new patients registered per month.
Pediatrician sees an average of 101 patients per week; internist sees an average of 82 patients per week; and family practitioners see an average of 118 patients per week.

Discussion Questions

1. What were the likely economic and political threats envisioned by the private practitioners in the establishment of the group? How could these be handled?
2. Assume management wishes to promote this expansion idea to the board of trustees. What additional information would be needed? Why? How would the case for expansion be presented?

NOTES

1. D.M. Kinzer, *Health Controls Out of Control: Warnings to the Nation from Massachusetts* (Chicago: Teach 'Em, 1977), p. 73.
2. D.F. Drake, "The Cost of Hospital Regulation," *Regulating Health Care: The Struggle for Control* ed. by A. Levin. Proceedings of the Academy of Political Science 33:4 (1980), p. 46.
3. Republican Health Plank, Congressional Quarterly 38:29 (July 19, 1980), p. 2035.
4. B. Biles, C.J. Schramm, J.G. Atkinson, "Hospital Cost Inflation Under Rate-Setting Programs," New Eng J Med 303:12 (Sept. 18, 1980), pp. 664-668.
5. Congressional Quarterly, Federal Regulatory Directory 1980-81 (Washington: Congressional Quarterly), p. 81.
6. State of Georgia, "General Budget Preparation Procedures, Fiscal Year 1977 Budget Development" in *Financial Management of Hospitals* ed. by H. Berman and L. Weeks (Ann Arbor: Health Administration Press, 1976), pp. 403-430.
7. J.D. Suver and R.L. Brown, "Where Does Zero Based Budgeting Work?" Harvard Business Review, 55:6 (Nov.-Dec., 1977), pp. 76-84.

Chapter 11

Temporary and Permanent Management Systems

Health care organizations are continually pressed to find solutions for problems and issues. Some problems are recurrent, and others are unique or occur at infrequent intervals. Those problems or issues that are recurrent often result in a more permanent management response, such as the establishment of personnel departments to meet the needs of organizations with high turnover or a rapidly expanding staff. On the other hand, management often needs simply a "helping hand" on some problem or issue for a short time, and a temporary management system comes into place.

TEMPORARY MANAGEMENT TECHNIQUES

Consultants

In general, consultants can be classified into four categories: (1) the individual entrepreneur consultant (the one-person show), (2) the health care consulting firm, (3) the general consulting organizations, and (4) the major national accounting and consulting firms.

The individual entrepreneur is a person who by reason of experience, expertise, glibness, or position is able to hang out a consultant's shingle and obtain clients. Oftentimes, such a person has developed a very narrow specialty and thus is invaluable to an organization having specific problems in that area. For example, there are people who make their living as hospital laundry consultants, telephone communication consultants, training consultants, or health maintenance organization (HMO) development consultants. University faculty are notorious for their consulting activities, most of which are short-time engagements in which an organization can pick a professor's brains for a fee.

Individual consultants have some important strengths, but they come with some built-in weaknesses. An obvious advantage is that the client is always dealing with the top person in the consulting organization and the very same person who will be doing the study and writing the report. Therefore, the client can continually monitor and evaluate the consultant's progress and, if necessary, the consultant can be redirected or fired. Perhaps even more important, it is easier to evaluate the expertise of an individual consultant than that of a firm prior to an engagement. A list of former clients and a check of those references, perhaps including a review of other reports prepared by the consultant, should indicate whether this is the person who should be engaged.

Of course, there are problems, too. First, there is no depth in a one-person organization. If the project's complexity is such that it requires additional expertise that the consultant does not possess, then this type of consultant either does a second-rate job on that component of the project or hires a "subcontractor" who may or may not satisfy the client. The second problem can come about when the organization is dealing with one of the "superstar" consultants or academic consultants and must share the consultant with other clients—which leads to the third problem. Academics who consult are also notorious for missing deadlines. If deadlines are important, then the individual's time commitments become an important factor in the selection. On the other hand, sometimes individual consultants are critical because of their political connections. For example, in one southern state it was well known that a particular retired government official turned consultant could expedite any certificate-of-need application.

Over the years a number of the individual consultants who have been particularly outstanding have developed specialty consulting firms in the health care field. The first generation of these firms was populated by former administrators (usually hospital administrators) who had established reputations for excellence. In general, they tackled a wide range of consulting type problems, and many of them established themselves as excellent "general practitioner" consultants. Because of their size, which often was in the area of 10 or 15 professionals, they offered a considerable breadth of services, but they rarely had depth in any specialty area other than something as generic as "planning" or "management development." To offset their weaknesses in depth, most of these firms have enough affiliations with independent consultants and sometimes academics so that special problems can be "subcontracted" with relative ease. Perhaps their major strength is their concentration on the health field; these firms are totally involved in the range of activities within health care. Thus, they bring to bear on any health care organizational problems a depth of historical and present knowledge of the health care system. Their solutions, or recommendations, to most problems can be expected to have the value of field trial, since they seldom work from theoretical models but rather have a pragmatic orientation based on experience.

More recently, the general management consulting firms and consulting groups of the large public accounting firms have entered the marketplace of health care consulting. The large national consulting firms have a depth of experience in the private and government sectors that can often be translated into solutions or recommendations for the health care industry. Also, because of their large size, they have a depth of knowledge that is simply not present in smaller firms. For example, some of these firms have subgroups that specialize in regulatory activities and can provide analytical expertise based on trends in other fields, as well as the health care field. The public accounting firms, some of which have been involved in health care for many years as auditors or financial advisers, have more recently expanded to take advantage of the opportunities in health care consulting. They provide financial feasibility studies, systems analysis, and the gamut of other management consulting. It could be said that the public accounting firms probably have the greatest strength in terms of work that is heavily financially oriented, the management consulting groups shine most in studies involving general management, and the health consulting groups are strongest in those areas where an in-depth understanding of the inner workings of a health care organization is required.

Another group of firms involved in consulting activity are the single specialty outfits that work in many fields, such as architectural, investment finance, and law firms. Many of these firms have gained enough experience in health care to offer themselves as consultants for problems in their specialized fields.

Consultants are needed basically because they have the time to do something clients want done but do not have the time to do or because they know something that clients need to know. Either way, clients are fundamentally buying time and expertise. The cost of the time is probably negligible if the consultants are doing something that has to be done. The problem is paying for time and not getting a satisfactory consultation. Thus, the issues are really, Does the consultant have the expertise to handle the client's needs, and what in fact are the client's needs?

In many health care organizations the needs are related to a specific problem or set of problems that have been recognized as serious enough to warrant attention by the top management and/or the board. Either management does not know enough about the possible solutions, or it does not have the time or inclination to work through the problem. For example, a number of states now require hospitals to have detailed five-year plans. Some institutions have chosen to give a presently employed staff person the responsibility for this plan. Others have hired new full-time planners, while a third group has turned to consultants. There is no one correct way to handle such a requirement—each organization must decide for itself which solution makes the best sense in light of its resources.

The critical points for the clients to remember are that they should begin by defining the consulting problem or problems for themselves. Second, they should interview as many as possible of the consultants and consulting firms that appear to have expertise in their area of concern. Third, they should carefully check references and review the previous work of the consultants. Fourth, they should find out as much as possible about the experience and expertise of those individuals who will be actually working on the job. Firms often send out their "top guns" to make the presentation and then have the actual work executed by much more junior and often inexperienced staff. Since most consultants are expensive, it is rather important to find out specifically who will be working on the project. Finally, the client should be prepared to give serious consideration to the consultant's findings—not necessarily adopt them automatically, but at least give them a fair chance.

Sometimes a hospital hires a consultant to buy time and credibility, not expertise. An outside consultant is sought to legitimize what is already known. If this is what is being considered, the manager must be careful to ensure that the consultant being engaged is in fact on the same wavelength. If not, the issues identified by the consultant are different from the issues previously identified by the client, and the net result is a report that recommends solutions not initially envisioned. In summary, clarity from the client's perspective about why a consultant is being used is likely to result in a set of decisions about hiring a consultant who can most expeditiously and expertly handle the engagement. Lack of clarity, on the other hand, results in disappointment for all concerned.

Teams—The Ad Hoc Committee and Task Force

The ad hoc committee and task force are temporary management structures in that they are set up for a special purpose, such as investigating an issue or developing strategies. The intent is that, after the committee or task force completes its mission, it will be disbanded. Many organizations have a more permanent structure through standing committees and special policy groups, such as an executive committee.

Is there a difference between a task force and an ad hoc committee? Probably not in any real substantive degree—they both exist for a limited period of time, they both have a narrow mission, and they both usually have multiple members, often from different parts of the organization. On an image level, which is sometimes transferred into substantive action, a committee appears to be a more deliberative and less action-oriented group, perhaps one that is more controlled by those in power than a task force. The image of a task force involves a sharply focused mission with high expectation for decisive action. Indeed, the task force notion almost envisions a military operation, such as an aircraft carrier with its destroyer escorts racing through the South Pacific heading toward a famous sea battle—with "Victory at Sea" music in the background.

Why bother with these task forces or committees? Management needs these systems for a variety of reasons, the most prevalent one being that a particular problem or issue has arisen and analysis of the problem requires a group effort. Management then assembles the group to do the job. Oftentimes, the problem has been clearly identified, and it appears that the solution has implications for many parts of the organization; in order to work with the various components on implementation, a team effort is necessary. Sometimes such an effort is developed simply to co-opt recalcitrant members of an organization. Another reason is to stall for time while management is looking for another solution. This can be observed particularly in government, where the response to a serious problem for which there appears to be no acceptable remedy is often to offer up to the public a blue-ribbon task force on the issue. This gives the illusion of action and decisiveness, while it buys time to be indecisive. This approach also allows individual managers to escape the flame for unpopular solutions to issues and problems. The task force has delivered the bad news, not management—management is now only implementing what the experts have decided.

There are a variety of problems with these temporary systems. An obvious one is that they are expensive, since they inevitably draw people in the organization away from their regular responsibilities. If members of the committee or task force are to be most effective in this temporary role, staff support must be provided, which is an additional expense. A second problem is that a great deal of time and energy must be expended in these groups just to make them a group. It takes time for the individuals to get to know one another and understand each other's strengths and weaknesses. Oftentimes, just as these groups appear to be coming together as teams, they are disbanded. Finally, a fundamental problem is that most people in management have not been socialized professionally to work as teams. It is often unclear who has what role, what each person's authority and responsibility are for the total team effort, and how they will be evaluated for their work on the project. The team will be effective in its mission to the extent that management can clarify the purpose of the committee and the scope of each member's authority and responsibility.

In health care organizations, this problem of roles and responsibilities is exacerbated because the notion of committees or task forces assumes a level of equality among the team members that does not exist outside of the meeting room. It is difficult to transcend those relationships simply because the group has been reassembled for a new purpose. The physician, nurse, administrator, and supervisor who relate to one another in a hierarchical manner outside of the task force find it difficult to relate in a consensual manner within a temporary management structure.

Finally, few people like feeling they have been "used." If it becomes obvious that the committee was a sham and was simply put together to be a smoke screen for something else (and the committee itself took its job seriously), or if the staff feel that they have been treated in a less than honest fashion by management and their opinions and analyses are not taken seriously, then lower morale and its consequences can be expected.

The Search Committee

As mentioned in Chapter 9, the search committee is becoming a popular ritual in virtually all but the smallest organizations. Usually, the search committee is put together for the purpose of filling a vacancy created by firing, resignation, or the development of a new position. The committee itself is not normally empowered to hire anyone, but rather is asked to recommend a person or several people to the next higher level where the decision will be made. Thus, the committee has the chore of recruiting and sifting but not the responsibility for the final decision. On the other hand, through its sifting process and recruitment strategy, it has a tremendous influence on the selection.

Search committees are usually put together to satisfy the internal constituencies of the organization and, to a lesser extent, to represent the organization to the outside world. As noted in the earlier chapter, search committees often buy time for management while it considers what to do about filling a position; they provide an image of a democratic process, which is certainly significant when an organization must comply with various government regulations on affirmative action; and a committee process assuages hostile constituencies. As with other committee structures, it also relieves managers of the responsibility for unpleasant decisions and gives them the clout to make the decisions they want to make.

The foregoing is clearly a cynical interpretation of the search committee and its functions. If management is to utilize search committees effectively, then certain principles must be followed. First, the committee must have adequate staff support so that its recruiting strategy can be properly implemented. For example, the committee should be able to develop an advertisement for the *New York Times* health care opportunity section and not have to place the ad personally and sort through the couple of hundred replies likely to be engendered. Later on in the process, the committee should be able to have letters prepared asking for references. Finally, committee members should know that their recommendations will be given the most serious consideration; and, if rejected, they will be given adequate explanations.

Part of their brief as they begin deliberations should be an investigation into the job itself. Does the organization really need the position? As part of this investigation, the search committee should conduct an exit interview with the person leaving so that the committee members can understand the nature of the job better. In certain instances, particularly when the job to be filled is a senior one or a very sensitive one, the committee should have access to consultants outside of the organization in order to get a better understanding of the position. For example, if a hospital is looking for a director of ambulatory care, talking to "successful" directors of ambulatory care would provide a better understanding of the skills and attitudes necessary for that position. In fact, the search committee should challenge the status quo of the organization and, through its efforts, implement the development plans of the organization.

Some search committees are very thorough. For example, when a small foundation was looking for a director, I was listed as a reference for one of the finalists. Not only did the chairman of the search committee spend about 30 minutes on the telephone discussing the candidate with me, he subsequently came to my office. During this three-hour discussion, the chairman learned a good deal about the candidate—and a good deal about me and what I did. Basically, he was appraising my "credibility" as a witness for assessing the candidate. At the University of Massachusetts the same process was followed with the search for a chancellor. After the final candidates were identified, teams of search committee members literally went to the home campus of the candidates and interviewed not only their superiors, but also their subordinates. From this emerged a picture, some say dossier, that allowed the committee to make its final recommendations.

These two examples must be contrasted with a number of examples in the health field when the board or a committee has been so impressed with a candidate that comprehensive analyses of their past experiences and references were not undertaken, and the net result was a disaster. The fit of the person to the organization is critical, and the use of a team to analyze that fit is beneficial—if the team is allowed to do its job.

PERMANENT MANAGEMENT TECHNIQUES

Quantitative Decision Making

Health care managers are constantly called upon to make decisions, and these decisions can be classified into three categories. In the first category are those decisions made when the manager totally understands all the factors that must be taken into account in the decision, as well as all the ramifications of any given decision. Despite the posturing of some managers that they are absolutely certain about what is happening, it is hard to conceive of a situation of such absolute certainty. The second category is the other end of the spectrum: total uncertainty. In these instances, decisions are made in a complete vacuum of information or are based on the implications of the decision. Again, it is difficult to find such decisions. Most decisions are in the third category; they are made under conditions of imperfect knowledge or risk. To some extent, then, almost all management decisions are calculated risks.

For horseplayers and managers, the chances of winning are considerably increased if there is greater knowledge upon which to make their decisions. In the past several decades, a host of new techniques and professions has been developed, all to help the manager make less risky (or more certain) decisions. In the past few years, the operations researchers have attempted to establish their hegemony over management decision making and have in part renamed their profession the management sciences—as if management were clearly more a science than an art.

One of the often mentioned criticisms of the operations researchers and management scientists has been that they tend to search for problems so that they can apply their techniques. Operational managers tend to operate in a rather different way; they have problems and look for ways of solving them. The interaction of the technique, solution, and political reality was well illustrated by the distinguished Columbia Professor E.S. Savas when he noted that "an algorithm which seems to prove the 'best' place for a drug treatment center is just down the block from a councilman's home, proves instead that the analyst is a poor one who should be ignored, or fired."[1] Indeed, the unconscious interests of an organization are seldom revealed on the first go-around of any decision process.

The gurus of the quantitative management processes are trained either in industrial engineering, operations research, or, more recently, the management and administrative sciences. Their commonality is a belief that decisions lend themselves to quantitative dissection, that what happens is logical, and that all of this can be explained mathematically. The tools of these trades tend to range from time and motion study to the more sophisticated techniques of simulations and model building. Typical of a quantitative technique is a decision matrix whereby probabilities are attached to possible alternative outcomes. Theoretically, the decision maker can then make the decision that is in the best interests of the organization.

The great value of quantitative decision making is that it forces the decision maker to make explicit what is most often implicit (and usually unclear). The techniques are great aids in the development of evidence for decision making. However, it must be recognized that the evidence is sometimes skewed by judgments, and care must be taken to examine the validity of those judgments before and not after a decision is made. Finally, the manager—much like a judge—must sift the evidence and then render a management decision that is in effect a judgment or opinion.

For the most part, the idea of trying to quantify decisions has apparently taken root in many health care organizations, but the most sophisticated techniques, such as decision matrices and simulations, are simply not being used. There are few organizations where such techniques are given much credence; in fact, even in an institution where operations researchers are on the staff and the top management is trained in these techniques, they are only used, as one senior executive noted, "for intellectual purposes—not real management.'' Although this technique is obviously in limited usage, it is classified here as a permanent technique because the next generation of health administrators have all received a double and sometimes triple dose of training in this technique, and they will expect to utilize it.

The academia-based management scientists are now realizing the weaknesses of their technique "in vivo," not only in the health field but also in industry. Within the next few years, the development of more realistic techniques that are in fact more useful for decision making can be expected, since one of the major ways in which providers can respond to the pressure from the government and third party payers is by better systems design and integration, smoother work flow, and higher productivity—all of which lend themselves to quantitative analysis.

Perhaps the potential "power" of the techniques and their possible limitations can best be illustrated by a typical problem facing health administrators and planners: locating a health facility. Selecting a location requires the analysis of a number of interacting variables; for example, the location and present as well as proposed future functions of neighboring facilities, the needs for services and beds in the community, and the probable utilization of the institution. Failure to account properly for any of these variables will probably cause the facility to be inappropriately utilized. How, then, does one go about locating a health facility so that it is most likely to be utilized by the population that it is planning to serve? Implicit in this question is the assumption that any given location of the facility will be better for some patients than others, that there will be fewer transportation and opportunity costs associated with going to the facility, and that, other conditions being equal, utilization will be greater when these costs have been minimized. This problem of health facility location to optimize an objective—in this instance, minimizing patients' cost—is conceptually similar to a typical industrial problem. A delivery firm tries to locate its warehouse so that delivery costs to a multitude of different clients with differing demands are minimized. In both cases, general demand patterns can be estimated, but the specific demands of a specific person cannot be predicted.

In solving this problem, a management scientist can apply a risk model devised for locating a warehouse to the problem of locating this facility. The assumptions explicit or implicit in this problem are that the number, location, and probable demand for medical care of the population can be estimated; that the demand is normally distributed; that the policy makers of the organization can decide what services are to be provided; that a probability statement can be attached to each service that will set a minimum level of service for each patient; and, finally, that the cost per mile per service can be estimated.

It appears reasonable that the number, location, and demand of the population can be determined, since census data can provide estimates of the population by age, sex, socioeconomic status, and location. The utilization estimates of the

National Center for Health Statistics can be used to extrapolate probable demand for the population.

Decisions made by institutional policy makers will provide information about the type of services (e.g., obstetrics, pediatrics, medicine, or surgery) that will be provided in the hospital. Also, these same policy makers will have to determine the probability of serving all the population all the time. In reality, the decision is not made as explicitly as it is called for in this problem; for example, when a board of trustees decides that a planned hospital will have a certain number of beds, it has implicitly made this judgment.

The next assumption is that demand for acute medical care among the various subsegments of the population, as measured by average length of stay or average number of visits to the physician, tends to be normally distributed. Is the population large enough to ensure these results? Without a large heterogeneous population, all of whom use the facility, this assumption may be open to question. Another way of considering this is, How are enough people "effectively enrolled" so that demand estimates can be made?

While it is reasonable to assume that the cost per mile per service can be measured, it is also a difficult figure to estimate. Included in such a figure must be overt costs—e.g., bus fares, gasoline, and parking charges—as well as opportunity costs. For example, the middle-aged individual who spends a day in the outpatient clinic is likely to lose some pay, while the retired individual is less likely to lose pay; hence, the opportunity costs for each are different.

Having set up the problem in this manner, the management scientist turns to a variety of mathematical formulas that result in a risk model and algorithm for its solution. Because of the extensive mathematics involved in solving this problem, the risk model, solution, and an illustration are presented in Appendix B.

What are the limitations of this approach? First and probably foremost is its "rationality." Implicit is the assumption that people act in a rational manner. Although it could be assumed that rational people would utilize those facilities that were less costly to them, evidence shows that people bypass more convenient facilities for a variety of reasons, such as familiarity with another institution. In spite of this known behavior, it is considered important to plan facilities rationally so that their location is functionally reasonable.

The second major limitation is the fact that variables other than minimizing cost to the patient enter into the selection of a site for a health facility. Zoning regulations, cost and availability of land, politics, and provider convenience are but a few of the important factors that, while possibly affecting the patient's bill, have little to do with the patient's overt and opportunity costs.

Even with these limitations, however, this approach does suggest a way in which known information in a community can be analyzed so that a service institution will have the highest likelihood of being utilized. Specifically, a developed model demonstrates that, when the objective is to minimize patient costs, the ideal locations are generally different for different mixes of services. In addition, one optimal location can provide a mix of different services with increased costs for some specific community members but probably with no additional cost for the community.

Secondly, with minor changes, a model could be used for locating the facility according to employee (rather than patient) cost. Such an objective might be realistically based on the problem of recruiting and retaining staff for an institution. If overt and opportunity costs for employees were less at one institution than another, other conditions being equal, it seems likely that individuals would work at the less costly (to them) institution.

Thus, using techniques developed for industry, a management scientist could help to clarify a problem and attempt to bring some degree of rational planning to health care. Limitations certainly exist—perhaps the main one is that, because of the relative lack of a competitive marketplace in health care, the economic considerations of the providers and consumers of health services are quite different from those of providers and consumers of other goods and services.

Marketing

Most health care provider organizations (with the exception of those that have had major fund-raising components, such as the Red Cross or Lung Association) have traditionally avoided "marketing." Indeed, they have had a practiced stance against "competitive" behavior and, except for cultivating relationships with likely generous benefactors, they have relegated marketing to a public relations function and turned it over to someone as an ancillary activity or utilized a "development" office. These attitudes and behaviors suggest a notion about health care that is to a large extent still prevalent; that is, the provision of health services is (or should be) removed from market forces and politics. It is a free enterprise mentality, but the consumer or public is simply not given the benefit of competition.

Much has changed in the past several years, and the idea of program and institutional competition has become a reality. The squeeze on resources of all types has meant that not every hospital can have the latest and fanciest piece of equipment or program. A decade or two ago, it seemed that every hospital in New York City had dreams of being a "teaching hospital" and was busily constructing its open heart surgical suite—although there were barely enough patients for a small fraction of these facilities. Today, building such units would require a level of community, professional, and financial support that was simply not part of the equation at that time.

Marketing, an often used technique in industry, is now starting to find favor in the health industry. It should be remembered that it is an old technique for which powerful tools have been developed; but, perhaps because of its "manipulative" image, it has been approached with doubt and great caution by those in the health field. Within the health care field, however, certain programmatic areas, particularly family planning, have already accumulated decades of invaluable field experience in consumer marketing techniques and strategies.

Marketing and health education are related and, to some extent, utilize similar techniques, but they approach the problem of consumer and professional behavior from somewhat different value orientations and perspectives. The health educator has tended to adopt the view that, if the consumers had better knowledge—that is, they could understand what was happening to them and why and/or they could understand what practices were expected of them—they would make the appropriate (right) choice. The marketer is more direct in urging a given choice and does not necessarily share the notion that more knowledge or practice information results in that choice being made; the approach may be at a less intellectual and more visceral level.

A comparison of the television commercials developed by the antismoking crusaders to those that had been given an award by the advertising fraternity because of their effectiveness illustrated this point. The message to the cigarette smoker was always pretty much the same—smoking stinks, it is lousy for the smoker's health, and it is dumb to smoke. Most smokers know that, but how can they break the habit? What are the cues for future action? On the other hand, Burger King's slogan, "Have It Your Way," indicated that the person who went to their restaurant would really be taken care of in a rather positive manner.

The cigarette advertisements in virtually any magazine are selling sex, power, class, and love. Those in the world of health care are not for the most part interested in selling sex, power, and love—although, to an extent, they are interested in presenting an image of "class," quality, and professional expertise and are supporting that image with substance. Kotler, in his useful book, *Marketing for Nonprofit Organizations,* defines marketing as "the analysis, planning, implementation and control of carefully formulated programs designed to bring about voluntary exchanges of values with target markets for the purpose of achieving organizational objectives."[2]

What are the markets for a typical not-for-profit health care organization? Figure 11-1 shows at least 16 important general markets that a health care organization is likely to be interested in communicating with and perhaps influencing. At various levels, government has power and, to some degree, discretion over the future course of the organization. It has ultimate authority through its fiscal controls, such as bonding authorities and rate reviews, and through approval mechanisms, such as the certificate-of-need process. In Massachusetts, the state legislators have played critical roles in the future of some hospitals by overriding the health planners and governor in order to approve the development of certain hospital projects that had been disapproved by the various health planning agencies. Without the continual involvement of the state legislators in the institution and

Figure 11-1 The Health Care Organization and Its Markets

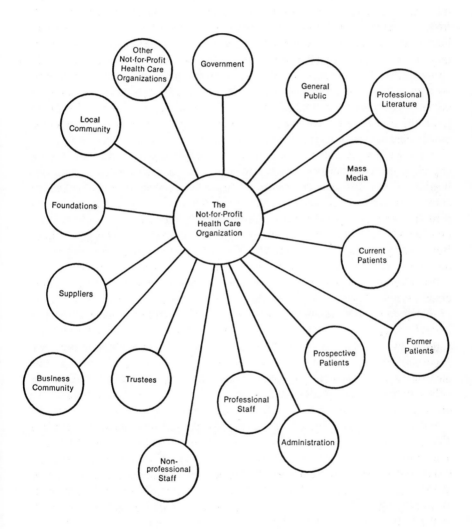

adequate marketing of the hospital's needs, it is unlikely that the planners' decisions would have been overridden.

The general public must always be considered a potential force for or against the organization. Most often they are quiet, but when an issue or concern arouses them they can be extremely vocal. For example, several years ago, the Harlem community was up in arms against the Health and Hospitals Corporation and the mayor over an incident in which a dietary employee and a medical resident had entered into an altercation over a napkin. More recently, community reaction has kept the Jewish Hospital of Brooklyn from being closed in spite of its bankruptcy. On a more positive side, in Hunterdon County, a relatively modest community, over 90 percent of the community donated funds to construct a new hospital—without the services of professional fund-raisers.

In any given health care organization, there are numerous professions represented, and numerous journals and publications relate to each of these professions. The literature represents recognition of both people and organizations. Professionalism in an organization is often enhanced when members of that organization identify with professional groups and when articles by them or about them and/or their programs are published in the professional literature. It is a level of recognition that is important and feeds the professional cycle.

The mass media are critical to the growth and survival of most organizations. Organizations need good press relations since, for the most part, the local newspapers, television stations, and radio stations provide a vital communications link within a community. The relationships here again are not built in a day or week but require careful nurturing on all sides.

Within any given program or institution there is a critical group that must be considered: current patients. These are the people currently going through the system, and they must be satisfied that the organization is functioning in their best interests. Together with the present patients, former patients will communicate their level of satisfaction or dissatisfaction to their friends and family. This will affect the various prospective patients, who will thus be inclined either to use the services of the organization or to find an alternative. Prospective clients can be "effectively enrolled" through a series of program workshops and other activities that get the person involved with the organization. As noted in earlier chapters, ambulatory care programs are ways in which hospitals get the general public in the habit of using their facility so that when they must be hospitalized they "know" where to go. Another way in which hospitals have begun to develop their relationships with the community is through educational programs, such as taped telephone messages that answer a range of health questions.

Within the organization itself there are constituencies that must be identified and "serviced." In Figure 11-1, administration is identified as a constituency; its needs must also be met if it is to be loyal and utilize its full efforts toward the welfare of the organization. Both the professional and nonprofessional staff must be cultivated as constituencies. If they have a positive attitude toward the organization, that attitude translates into a positive behavior. Staff who are unconcerned with how the organization is perceived or functions are simply ambassadors and communicators of ill will to other constituencies. Physicians, for example, who are displeased with a hospital or even uncertain as to what is occurring in the institution and their own place in the developing organization, often show their feelings of vulnerability by expressing open hostility or even by moving their patients into other facilities. A management that is sensitive to the needs of this constituency and tries to secure their involvement in the organization's development is more likely to retain the loyalty of these people. Trustees—present, past, and potential—are a group with a special interest in an organization and should be recognized as a special constituency.

Also, there are many potentially important groups outside of an organization, some of whom the organization is presently doing business with and others whom it is likely to do business with in the future, to whom marketing activities would be important. The business community is always an important source of general and sometimes specific support; from this group often come trustees, donations, and other types of support. Suppliers, for example, are people who are in a direct financial relationship with an organization. If they understand the nature of an organization's work, they are more likely to view favorably its needs for special attention.

Private foundations can also be considered a constituency for the not-for-profit organization. These foundations are often a source of financial and spiritual support for the development of new and innovative programs or the support of less innovative but important on-going programs.

Marketers utilize various techniques. Usually when marketing comes to mind, people think first of advertising. With the exception noted earlier, advertising has not been a major tool for health care organizations. On the other hand, almost $500 million per year is being spent on marketing activities directed toward the health field. Indeed, in a recent issue of the *American Journal of Public Health*, there were 16 advertisers, including 7 drug companies and 4 publishers. In an issue of *Hospitals, The Journal of the American Hospital Association*, there were 100 advertisers, including medical equipment firms, public utilities, proprietary hospital groups, clothing manufacturers, drug companies, investment finance firms, and suppliers of materials ranging from paper to x-rays.

On September 1, 1977, the *New York Times* carried a story on the American Hospital Association's guidelines for hospital advertising. The article noted that the association felt there were five legitimate purposes for advertising: "public education about available services, public education about health care, accounting to the community, seeking support, and employee recruitment." The guidelines themselves call for "truth and accuracy, fairness, no comparisons, no claims of prominence and no promotion of individual professionals." Hospitals have often used newspaper advertising as a way of delivering their annual reports or occasionally raising funds. Several years ago, the Duke Medical Center in Durham, North Carolina, placed an entire section of advertising in the Sunday edition of the *New York Times* as a mechanism to raise money for its new medical center.

On a less ambitious and less costly level, health care organizations often publish "house organs." These in-house newspapers tend to focus on the internal constituencies and are intended primarily to promote the institution and its staff. They generally include many photographs of buildings and important people. If there is one criticism of these newspapers, it is that they tend to look for such a large audience that they lose everyone. For example, some newsletters seem to be filled with endless gossip columns from various staff groups; much of the material is self-generated and therefore self-serving. The front page may be devoted to a new CAT scanner the institution has bought and may show a picture of the radiology chief and a trustee inspecting the CAT scanner. Who is the audience? No one can be satisfied, and some might argue no one then will be dissatisfied. Perhaps it is time for some larger organizations to start publishing multiple organs targeted at different audiences. Through this example, two points should be considered. What is it that the organization wants to communicate? To whom does it want to communicate its messages?

One approach is that the health care organization knows what its public needs and must simply find the right vehicle for communication. Another approach is that the health care organization thinks it knows what it wants to communicate and the needs of its constituencies but engages in market research to find out with greater precision what those needs are. Analysis of past demand for services, attitude and behavior surveys, and test marketing are some of the ways the health care organization can define its targets. Once the targets are in focus, advertising, direct mail, or a range of other techniques can be used. A few years ago, a psychiatric hospital found out through a series of interviews that it had an image in the community as a hospital for rich, crazy people and that most people, including potential referral sources, were unaware of the scope of their services and the seriousness of their teaching commitments. Further, few people realized that they were more than willing to take indigent patients. After research had uncovered these problems, the hospital's management went into action with brochures, an information hot line, direct letters to referral agencies, and personal meetings.

Marketing problems are easily mishandled. Exhibit 11-1, for example, shows an announcement that was sent to students and staff at Columbia. What is the message of this card? It appears that people who can or are willing to diagnose themselves as psychoneurotic (whatever that is) might be seen. Perhaps if the message were more personalized on a direct mail piece (easily done in these days of the automatic typewriter) and addressed students about anxiety related to starting or returning to college, problems with interpersonal relationships, or depression about the future, while addressing faculty in terms which they could

Exhibit 11-1 Card Announcing Psychoanalytic Services

The Columbia University Psychoanalytic Clinic for Training and Research is prepared to offer intensive long-term psycho-analytic therapy to suitable patients with psychoneurotic disorders, psychosomatic illnesses, problems of childhood and of early adulthood.

Questions may be referred to the Director of the Clinic at 927-5000.

John J. Weber, M.D.
Ms. Rosalind Chambers, Administrative Assistant

relate to ("Worried about tenure?"), the response might have been greater. In fact, in this instance, they did develop a more personalized approach to their potential markets and at last report were more successful in attracting clients.

In essence then, marketing is based on the assumptions that all constituencies make choices at least at some levels and that these choices can to some degree be influenced. There is competition among health care organizations; and, although a marketing strategy may not involve direct comparisons with other organizations, it does involve indirect comparisons. The successful marketer communicates well and has a good product. One person whose mother had died in a large teaching hospital received a patient opinion poll a few days after the death. He did not fill it out because he felt the service and the attitudes of the staff were so poor that either management was incompetent or simply did not care. When patients or their families feel that the organization is so unresponsive, then communications may not be too useful and, in some instances, may be offensive.

Marketing then is targeted communication that requires the communicator to listen effectively to the needs of those they wish to communicate with and to respond in a manner that can be understood by the target audience.

Organizational Development

Organizational development (or OD as it is popularly referred to) is concerned with behavior and attitudes within organizations. The idea is that many things can be manipulated within an organization so that it can more efficiently and effectively meet its goals. OD includes a wide range of techniques that can be applied not only to the staff of an organization but also to the organization itself. For example, OD specialists often focus their energy on identifying, clarifying, and sometimes changing the goals of the organization. To some extent then, OD is concerned with conditioning an organization to deal with the stress of a changing world (at the most general level) and a changing need and demand for the organization's present line of services (at a microlevel).

While the quantitative analysis of problems has for the present attracted the expertise of operations researchers, mathematicians, and engineers, the world of OD has attracted a different group of people. These people might be classified as the behavioral scientists, since they come from the ranks of sociologists, psychologists, and social psychologists. While some writers trace OD back to sensitivity training, in which great emphasis was placed on training all levels of staff to understand their own needs, others' needs, and the organization's needs, the history of management is full of attempts to develop organizations in such a way that they would function more efficiently and effectively and be better conditioned for change. For example, the utopian communities of the mid-1800s had an element of OD in them. The Northampton Association of Education and Industry was a group that owned a silk factory, a farm, a lumber mill, and other enterprises. It organized itself so that it had shorter work hours than was the tradition of the time, healthier living conditions, and better food than was available to most workers during that period. While there were moral reasons for the organization, there were also economic reasons. Each member worked at a task that was "theoretically suited to his tastes and talents."[3] Even the frequently maligned Fredrick Winslow Taylor, whose interest in "scientific management" caused him to classify iron workers in rather uncomplimentary terms, can in some respects be considered an OD person, although in a rather coercive way.[4] He wanted to push (some might argue kick) people into producing; the latter day OD specialists want to lead employees into producing. The world of Theory Y then is that of the OD staff, and many techniques noted earlier are within their area of interest: participative management, job enrichment, sensitivity training, and leadership development.

Whether an organization has decided to develop a formal OD program or not, the elements of a program exist, e.g., the reality of how well that organization functions on a day-to-day basis and how well it responds to the demands of change. The problem for management is first to understand what is happening. How does it go about understanding its organizational health status?

A typical way of finding out what is happening is through survey "research." Research in most organizations ranges from elegant experimental designs to less elegant back-of-the-envelope inquiries. To the extent that an organization can afford it, formal research should be undertaken. The results of the research should be not only reliable and valid but also reproducible—rerunning the research should produce similar findings—and the research should provide the information needed. An example of the problem with survey research is the hospital patient opinion poll in which a form is sent to patients after their discharge from the institution to ask for their opinion on a range of matters:

How would you rate the admissions process?
    Too slow. Too fast. Just right.
How was the food?
    Good. Bad. So-so.

What is the problem with these polls? First, a very small percentage of discharged patients respond, and very little is known about those patients who do respond. The respondents may not accurately reflect the population that utilizes the institution.

Within an organization, surveys of staff may be viewed with considerable suspicion. Several years ago, a survey of faculty at Columbia University was undertaken in order to establish workload standards. The reason for the survey was known, and the response from the faculty indicated that virtually everyone was putting in 80-hour workweeks—a finding about which there might be some legitimate doubt.

Another mechanism for developing evidence about what is occurring in the organization is the analysis of data that are routinely collected by the organization. For example, within an organization data are normally collected about the number of people hired and fired each month and the number of those who resign voluntarily. These data should be translated into labor turnover figures that can be studied for trends. The quality of staff recruited can be an indication of many things, such as changes in the marketplace or changes in the perception (and reality) of the organization. Teaching hospitals often rate themselves on the number of residency positions they fill and the quality of their residents.

Production data are useful if reviewed on a continual basis and analyzed for trends—including negative production, such as employee grievances. What are the grievances about? How frequently do they occur, and to what extent are they limited within a certain group of staff or supervisory personnel? Such information indicates which parts of the organization are experiencing the greatest strain and, to an extent, how that strain is being resolved. Some strain simply is not going to surface, however, and continual probes must be made in order to find out not only what is happening but also what is likely to be happening.

Comparisons with similar organizations are useful. Administrators do not usually rush into innovation; rather, they ask what others have experienced with such innovations. Such comparisons among health care organizations, particularly hospitals, are relatively available because of services such as the professional activity survey and the hospital activity survey. Both of these services, the former offered by the Commission on Professional and Hospital Activities in Ann Arbor, Michigan, and the latter offered by the American Hospital Association in Chicago, Illinois, provide organizations with mean, median, and standard deviation data on a range of professional and administrative services. Thus, organizations can see whether their length of stay for a certain procedure is out of line; in the same way, they can compare their food service costs.

At a very pragmatic level, health care organizations can, to some extent, see how they are doing in the marketplace. Are consumers interested in utilizing their services? Does a family planning service that wants to serve people from all socioeconomic classes have a clientele only of poor people? Does a neighborhood health center that is calling for financial independence of government grants have the ability to attract full-paying clients? To what extent is its present patient load made up of people who can be converted into full-paying patients? Readers of the *New York Times* who during 1979 read numerous stories about the "downfall" of the Jewish Hospital of Brooklyn might not remember that less than a quarter of a century earlier the Jewish Hospital had been one of the premier teaching hospitals in New York, with an international reputation for many of its efforts, such as its pioneering work in open heart surgery. Health care organizations are vulnerable to shifts in preference by patient and physician consumers—an important lesson to remember.

Change must be considered almost inevitable within any organization. The manager's problem is to organize that change. Some change is obvious; everyone expects it and can deal with it. While effecting that type of change takes a great deal of time and energy, it is not likely to be disruptive to the organization. On the other hand, much of what occurs in an organization is hard to see and even harder to manage. How can management shake the lethargy from an organization that considers itself stable and steady, even though the world around it is changing rapidly and eroding its base? How could 17 hospitals in New York City find themselves bankrupt in the mid-1970s? How could well-known teaching institutions with top flight management go out of business? How did W. T. Grant or, more recently, Sears Roebuck and Chrysler make such massive miscalculations that they led to bankruptcy court in the first instance and great difficulties in the others?

OD calls for management through attention to clear objectives, the catch phrase being management by objectives; job enrichment, i.e., more concern for the cerebral activities associated with a job than the mechanical or labor activities; and, as noted earlier, a heightened level of sensitivity. As the next few years unfold, many new techniques will emerge. The value of any of these techniques will be increased or mitigated by the ability of an organization to understand both where it is and where it wants to go.

An analogy to OD might be the stress test electrocardiogram. A regular electrocardiogram reveals how well the heart is functioning at a resting time, but the stress test measures the heart's performance under conditions of duress. To the extent that a person is in good condition, the heart can perform well. Organizations need to do two things: first, they must develop programs to get into condition; second, they must periodically take their electrocardiogram to measure their health status.

One hospital in central Pennsylvania and one in New Mexico have done this. Several years ago, they set up small Health Maintenance Organizations (HMOs). Both hospitals expected the HMOs to be deficit operations, but they were willing to develop them. Why? Their view was that the HMO or some variant on the basic theme of prepaid group practice was likely to be a major component of medical care in the 1980s. Before it was imposed on them, the hospitals wanted to try a small scale experiment and see what they could learn. In a sense, they were test marketing the HMO both externally, to see how it functioned outside of their hospitals, and internally, to see its implications for the rest of their systems. The projects were undertaken by these hospitals to prepare their organizations for important transitions that they are now likely to face in a better condition.

CASE STUDY

Green Memorial Hospital*

The search firm visited the hospital for several days; met with key members of the medical staff, board, and administration; and made the following tentative conclusions:

- Green Memorial is a good quality community hospital.

- The newer practitioners (almost 40 percent have moved into the area in the past ten years) are extremely well trained and committed to Green.

- The medical staff view administration as acceptable and dull. They want to see the hospital improve in a qualitative way—but without establishing a teaching program.

---

*Continued from case study in Chapter 9.

- The board is dominated by the chairman, and the rest of the members are poorly informed of activities and lethargic.

- Competition from other hospitals is limited, and relationships with the Health Systems Agency are good, although trouble with the regulatory agencies is anticipated in the future.

- The hospital's financial picture is good. Occupancy is at the 91 percent level, and for the past four years the hospital has had an excess of revenues over expenses of more than $175,000 per year.

- The top management group is too thin; in addition to a chief executive officer, there should be at least two assistant administrators. The search firm found no major objection to the corporate reorganization recommended by the consultant.

- The middle management ranks (department heads) were found to be uneven. The finance/accounting person was viewed as weak because of his limited expertise and lack of interest in developing computerized management information systems. The departments of nursing, personnel, and food service were viewed as fair, and the clinical ancillary services, such as radiology, laboratory, pharmacy, and physical therapy were viewed as excellent.

- The search firm felt that the chief executive officer position for this hospital should pay approximately $45,000 plus a package of fringe benefits worth approximately $12,000.

Exhibit 11-2 Sample Resumé

John J. Astor
817 Back Bay Road
Boston, MA

Education
1970   Harvard University
(Ph.D.)   School of Public Health
              Dissertation: A Mathematical Model To Establish
              Determinants of Physician Behavior in Commu-
              nity Hospitals

1965   Johns Hopkins School of Public Health
(M.P.H.)   Concentration: Public Health Administration

1963   Princeton
(A.B.)   Major: Mathematics
              Minor: Political Science

Employment
1978 to date Private Consultant
              Boston, MA

1976-1978   Vice President for Planning
              Hospital Council of Long Island

1970-1976   Assistant Professor
              University of Utah
              School of Public Health
              Department of Health Administration

1965-1967   Assistant Administrator
              Calvin Coolidge Hospital
              Cummington, Maine

Publications
Books
1974   The Dynamics of Community Hospitals
              (N.Y.: Viva Press)

Exhibit 11-2 continued

1977   Trends and Perspectives in Community
                   Hospital Administration
                   (Boston: Big Green & Co.)

Articles (This list includes only articles published since 1979—a list
of the 43 previous articles is available upon request.)

"Disaster Planning in a Community Hospital,"
Hospital Planning, XI (April, 1979), pp. 11-15.

"Construction Management in Hospital Renova-
tion Projects," *International Journal of Construction Management* 17 (July, 1979), pp. 23-25.

"Fire Department Hospital Relations," *The
Firefighters Almanac* (Aug. 1979), p. 41.

"The Mathematics of Hospital Administration,"
Journal of Mathematical Hospital Administration
75 (Dec. 1979), pp. 91-114.

"Technology in Hospital Housekeeping," *Update*
X (March, 1980), pp. 77-83.

Memberships

Fellow - American College of Hospital Administration
Fellow - American Public Health Association
Member - Harvard Club

Personal

DOB April 19, 1940
Divorced - 3 children

Exhibit 11-3 Sample Resumé

Clark Kent, F.A.C.H.A.
Administrator
Smallville Hospital
Smallville, New Jersey
Telephone (201) 314-0100

Personal Data:

Born Nov. 14, 1920 Krypton Township, N.J.
Married June 11, 1950 to Lois Lane Kent
  Three children: Clark 4/1/54
                 Perry 1/14/56
                 Lana 9/30/60

Professional Chronology

1938-1942	University College of Journalism State College, N.J.
1942-1945	U.S. Army (1st Lt. Signal Corps)
1945-1947	Newspaper Reporter
1947-1949	Graduate Student in Hospital Administration Columbia University, N.Y.C. Awarded M.S. in Hospital Administration. Residency at Brooklyn Eye and Ear Hospital
1949-1955	Assistant Administrator St. Paul's Hospital Cleveland, Ohio

Exhibit 11-3 continued

1955-1960	Associate Executive Director University Medical Center Richmond, Virginia (A 700-bed university teaching hospital)
1960-1965	Executive Director University Medical Center Richmond, Virginia
1965-1972	Medical Group Manager Cartersville Medical Center Cartersville, N.Y. (An 18-physician private group practice)
1972-date	Administrator Smallville Hospital Smallville, N.J. (A 150-bed medical school affiliated teaching hospital)

Exhibit 11-4 Sample Resumé

Anne Rogers Fineman

Office

Department of Health Services
City of New York
125 Worth St.
New York City
(212) 490-4000

Home

118 W. 72 Street
New York, NY
(212) 781-0059

Present Position (Since Jan. 1979)

Deputy Commissioner
Department of Health Services
New York City

From July 1976 to Jan. 1979

Vice Chairman and Professor
Department of Community Medicine
University Hospital of University Medical College
Richmond, Virginia

From June 1975 to July 1976

White House Fellow
Washington, D.C.

From June 1970 to June 1975

Assistant (then) Associate Professor
Department of Community Medicine
Medical College of Cleveland
Cleveland, Ohio

Exhibit 11-4 continued

Residency Training in Family Practice at the Queenstown Medical Center, Queenstown, Ohio.

Publications (as of 1979)

Three textbooks in community medicine
Twenty-four articles

Note: Complete list available on request.

Military Experience

Three years (1967-1970) as Naval Medical Officer. Trained as flight surgeon.

Exhibit 11-5 Sample Resumé

Mary Ann Smith
Associate Director
Cleveland Community Hospital
Cleveland, Oregon
(913) 477-0101

Job Objective: To be the chief executive officer of a medium-sized
community hospital.

Professional Experience

1977-date	Associate Director, Cleveland Community Hospital. This is a 419-bed nonteaching hospital. Responsibilities involve administrative direction of nine clinical and nonclinical departments.
1975-1977	Assistant Administrator, Veterans Administration Hospital, Port Jefferson, Oregon. This is a 1000-bed teaching hospital. Responsibilities involved administrative direction of five nonclinical departments.
1970-1975	Assistant Administrator, Kaiser Hospital, Petersburg, Washington. This is a 145-bed HMO affiliated hospital. Responsibilities involved planning and direction of 20-bed expansion and seven clinical and nonclinical departments.
1968-1970	Administrative Resident Green Memorial Hospital

Exhibit 11-5 continued

1962-1966	Bachelor of Arts Student
	University of Illinois
	Major: Sociology

Fellow	American College of Hospital Administrators
Nominee	Young Hospital Administrator of the Year (1974)
Member	Cleveland Area HSA Board

Home Address

1717 Town Road
Burlington, Oregon
(913) 549-1317

Exhibit 11-6 Sample Resumé

John Doe
1420 Quentin Road
Brooklyn, N.Y.
(212) 712-3456

D.O.B. 12/11/30

Education:

New York University	(1951) B.S. Accounting
Pace College	(1955) M.S. Business Management

Professional Experience

1951-1957	Auditor, Assistant Manager Kris and Kringle (C.P.A. Firm) New York City
1957-1964	Assistant Comptroller Orange Community Hospital
1964-1969	Comptroller Orange Community Hospital
1969-1975	Assistant Director for Finance Orange Community Hospital
1975-Date	Consultant John Doe Associates

Personal: Divorced (2 children)
No military service (exempt because of asthma)

Discussion Questions

1. The candidates whose resumés are shown in Exhibits 11-2 through 11-6 are on the firm's "short list." In view of the needs of the hospital, what is each candidate's suitability for the chief executive officer position?
2. What criteria should be used?
3. What questions are raised by the resumés of each of the candidates?
4. Who would be the top two choices? Why?

NOTES

1. E.S. Savas, "New Directions for Urban Analysis," *Interfaces*.
2. P. Kotler, *Marketing for Nonprofit Organizations* (Englewood Cliffs, NJ: Prentice-Hall, 1975), p. 5.
3. H.H. Davis, "The Northampton Association of Education and Industry," in *The Northampton Book* (Northampton, MA: The Tercentary Committee, 1954), p. 109.
4. F.W. Taylor, *The Principles of Scientific Management* (New York: Harper and Brothers, 1911).

Chapter 12

Strategic Planning

Planning does not always work, as can be seen in the experience of the Ford Motor Company with the Edsel; the headline-making bankruptcies of Penn Central and W.T. Grant; and the fiscal disasters of Lockheed, Chrysler, and Rolls Royce. All of these corporations had in common worldwide reputations—large organizations with seasoned executives and talented planners—but they failed. They failed because the marketplace is so complex; matching the demand for services or products to needs while considering competition, availability, economic conditions, and myriad other factors requires almost perfect planning (if that exists). A slight miscalculation can spell organizational disaster.

In the health care field, for the past several generations it has appeared that the demand for services and the money to finance the services have been unlimited. Controls on services were essentially unknown until a few years ago. For the most part, the free enterprise mentality still makes it difficult to provide comprehensive regulation in the health industry. Any surgeon, for example, can simply begin to practice in any community without regard to the needs of that community for another surgeon. Critics of the U.S. health system attribute the high surgery rates throughout the United States to such situations and to the overabundance of surgeons.

How are hospital beds distributed? Who shall say when and where a new facility will be built? Perhaps the most glaring example of the lack of real control in this area is the Naval Hospital in New Orleans. The federal government ignored its own planning agencies and alleged fiscal concerns and built a naval hospital in honor of the former head of the House Armed Forces Committee, Congressman F. Edwin Hebert. The hospital was built on a Naval Reserve facility that was practically closed in a community where there were practically no naval or other armed forces activities. In fact, at the time the Navy was busy planning the hospital, the federal government was busy trying to close the neighboring U.S. Public Health Service Hospital for a variety of reasons, one of which was underutilization. Eventually, the Naval Hospital was built at a cost in excess of $100 million, opened, and so underutilized that within a few years it was leased to a community hospital corporation.

The U.S. health system contrasts sharply with that of Great Britain, where centralized planning is a critical component of the National Health Service. For example, physicians cannot simply move into any community, set up practice, and receive payment from the government. They must move into an open area, essentially receiving authorization to practice in that community from the government, before they can be reimbursed for National Health Service patients. Specialists must find an authorized post at an authorized hospital, or, once again, they will receive no fees from the government. Of course, British physicians who decide to be totally private entrepreneurs and not accept patients who will not pay privately can practice anywhere they choose, but this occurs in relatively few instances. Under the British scheme, physicians can be distributed according to the population's needs rather than the physicians' needs. In the United States, the distribution is made primarily on the basis of the physicians' needs.

Strategic planning is primarily concerned with an organization's need to survive and flourish in a competitive, often quagmire-like environment. In one sense, it is a subset of general planning; but, because of the "future shock" that most health care organizations are going through with seemingly simultaneous breathtaking breakthroughs in technology and regulation, strategic planning has come to occupy center stage for many health care organizations. Steiner has defined strategic planning as "the process of deciding the basic mission of a company, the objectives which it seeks to achieve and the major strategies and policies governing the use of resources at the disposal of the firm to reach its objectives."[1]

It should be emphasized that planning is an integral function of all management—and at all levels—and not simply a function that is delegated to a special group of people labeled planners. Indeed, Steiner suggests that in an "ideal" situation in an "average" company, the chief executive officer should be spending more than half his or her time planning for more than two years ahead. At the department manager level, he suggests that such advance planning should involve closer to five percent of the manager's time, but a significant portion of the manager's time should be involved with time horizons of less than six months. Planning is an activity that requires a synthesis of virtually all the skills within an organization, and strategic planning involves the probing analysis of organizational objectives, strengths, and (most sensitively) weaknesses. Since "a cardinal purpose of planning is to discover future opportunities and make plans to exploit them," it is almost a necessity of organizational life to undertake these planning efforts on a continual basis.[1]

There are inherent difficulties in the process of strategic planning. Problem number one is: who does it? Theoretically, it ought to be an organizational effort. Since strategy and tactics are involved, however, the senior management staff (and sometimes just the chief executive officer) often take the responsibility for strategic planning. As was noted earlier, it is easy to get caught up in the dynamics of the day-to-day running of the organization and not set aside the "ideal" planning time. In fact, a common criticism of strategic planning is that the senior executives do not give it sufficient thought, which leads to the second problem: continuity. To be successful, a strategy must have a certain element of continuity; otherwise, the organization that is to implement the strategy is likely to provide more of a hindrance than a help in the implementation.

Strategic planning requires an enormous amount of information and data. The subproblems here, of course, are the availability, timeliness, and quality of information. For example, how does an ambulatory care program determine the potential demand for its services? Census data are usually out-of-date, and it is difficult to get straight answers from physicians about their practices. Without actually undertaking an expensive and time-consuming survey, management is effectively forced to rely on informed guesses.

A final problem to be noted is: who shall evaluate the strengths and weaknesses of the organization? The analysis of the strengths is always a pleasant and usually self-serving job, but what about the weaknesses? How does management say that the institution is losing its patient base because of a move to the suburbs that had been vehemently opposed by the board chairman? In less dramatic terms, it might be asked, How many organizations ever sit back to analyze their success? Or, for that matter, to what extent do they understand what success is for their organizations? In business organizations success usually refers to the "bottom line" or profit. An organization that cannot produce a profit is an organization that simply must leave the marketplace. In health care organizations, other than the few proprietary ones, the measure of success has never been profit—but what has it been? Prestige is one of the intangibles that health care organizations have striven toward, as well as technical excellence. To some extent, survival has been a major goal in the last few years; while society is not asking many of its charitable organizations to make a profit, it certainly is saying "Stop losing so much money."

The last decade has seen a spate of hospital bankruptcies in New York City. One large teaching hospital had an endowment so large that in 1960 the endowment income represented approximately 20 percent of its operating budget. By 1975, only 15 years later, despite a growth in the endowment and its earnings, the budget had increased five times and the endowment income now represented less than 10 percent of the budget. All during this time, the hospital had the same management team; over the 15 years, the team had not increased in size, breadth, or depth. In fact, it was attempting to run the institution the same way as it had for 15 years. The managers were caught up in the mystique of their own making about the greatness and invulnerability of their institution. Finally, the chief executive officer retired, a new person was brought in, and the proverbial "house of cards" started to fall.

On one hand, health care organizations must deal with a mystique about what they do; on the other hand, they must consider some realities, such as a payroll that must be met.

To complicate these basic considerations, health care organizations must consider their role as socially responsible organizations. These responsibilities have many dimensions; for example, they have a responsibility toward the overall financial well-being of the nation; toward patients, medical staff, and personnel employed by the organization; and toward the community. The Mary Imogene Bassett Hospital in the small upstate New York town of Cooperstown took upon itself an interesting social responsibility. It has (or at least until a few years ago had) the only food service facility in the area that was open to the public 24 hours a day. In the early hours of the morning, not only were the late night workers at the hospital, but also a range of others, including local police and late night party-goers. According to the hospital's administrator, the hospital felt a special responsibility toward their community, and the opening of their cafeteria was one way in which they met that responsibility.

A more dramatic example comes from a New Jersey hospital that was in the process of closing down patient rooms because of a decline in census. In the interest of good management, such cutbacks would normally result in staff layoffs. In this case, however, there were no layoffs because the hospital was concerned about the economic implications to its community if 100 people were unemployed. Here again can be seen the reality facing the health care organization; it is both a social organization, with special responsibilities because of what it does as its everyday work, and an economic organization, with a vast influence on the total economic system because of the resources it commands. The point is emphasized by the fact that, in many parts of the United States, health services may be the largest industry in town.

To this point then, an organization interested in strategic planning would have considered a range of basic issues, such as what its definition of success was, what its view of its social responsibility might be, and, most importantly, what its objectives were. In the business sense, this would answer the fundamental question, What business are we in and why?

The next step in management's strategic planning is to understand what is occurring in the environment around the organization and how it is likely to affect the organization. Environmental changes can be classified into broad categories, such as technological changes, social and political changes, and economic changes. The health field is one that has become particularly sensitive to technological change. Consider how drug therapy has affected the mental health field, literally emptying hospitals and restoring people to the community. Perhaps an even more dramatic example is the essential elimination of the tuberculosis sanitarium and, for all practical purposes, the elimination of tuberculosis itself. Organizations dedicated to that disease, whether they were fund-raising or service delivery, needed to change their mission in order to survive. Some did; for example, the tuberculosis associations became lung associations. Others, such as the Will Rogers Sanitarium in Saranac Lake, New York, did not, and they closed. Considering the research priorities and great financial investment that is being made primarily by the government, is it so unlikely that within the next 10 or 20 years cancer will be eliminated and heart disease and stroke will be controlled? Such changes would have a profound impact on virtually any health care organization—but how many have considered such eventualities?

The development of computers that allow for the storage and transmittal of vast amounts of information has had an equally significant effect on the health system. In his book *Five Patients,* Michael Crichton talks about a patient at Logan Airport being examined by a physician at Massachusetts General Hospital, several miles and a river away.[2] If a few miles, why not a thousand? Television and satellites are making all of this possible. Perhaps the physician distribution problem will be solved with television studios, telemetric equipment, and physicians on duty in emergency studios equipped with monitors and computers.

The technological developments of other fields also find their way into the health system. Surgeons are beginning to trade their old steel scalpels for laser knives that "cut cleaner and faster." It was not so long ago that the glass syringe and needle that was sent to central supply for sharpening gave way to disposable plastic syringes and needles that cut down the problems of infections (and some say dull needles). Whether all of these changes are progress or not is probably a debatable point, but health care organizations must be sensitive to these possibilities.

Because of the great dependence of most health care organizations on people, both as patients and providers, and on the government as a source of financing, social and political changes greatly affect these organizations. For example, demographic trends, such as suburbanization, population mobility, and increased levels of education, all have an impact on the health system. It has been demonstrated in some research that population mobility has resulted in greater utilization of the emergency room by the physicianless patient. Some suggest that the depersonalization of our society has increased litigation. For the health field, this has resulted in an increase in malpractice claims and a subsequent rise in premiums, which eventually is translated into higher fees. As one of the three largest employers in the United States, the health system is faced with hiring people who are significantly better educated than their parents and with offering them more challenging jobs.

Unionization in the health care field, not only among unskilled and skilled "hourly" workers but also among the professionals, can also be viewed as part of a social trend in labor relations that is part of a larger social movement of civil rights. The effect of social and political changes on the health system can be seen in the changes that took place during the 1970s over the issue of abortions. For the first time in U.S. history, an abortion could be performed as a legal procedure. Some hospitals spent years delaying the offering of this service; others simply refused to offer it. Recently, in western Massachusetts, the fact that one hospital offered abortion services was a key issue blocking a merger of two facilities. Subsequently, the payment for abortions under Medicaid affected the availability and distribution of services and manpower.

It now appears that the health system is fully immersed in an era of economic changes that affect it. One of the chief causes of inflation in the United States, some argue, is the health industry. Opposing groups bring out impressive charts to support their positions but, an industry that is so large and consumes such a significant portion of federal monies would obviously be part of the problem and an area to be scrutinized in the search for a solution. In the past, the health care field has been almost a sacred cow, and to cut a health budget was close to unacceptable. Clearly, those days are over and health services must compete with all other activities for money. The health system must live in and be affected by the general economic climate. Inflation or the increased cost or unavailability of energy affects all the components of the health system.

In the last generation or so, traditional philanthropic sources for health facilities have dried up, and health care organizations have been forced to seek public and private funding for their operations. The notion of a hospital administrator on Wall Street signing a prospectus for a tax-exempt bond offering would have been absurd not too many years ago, but today it is a reality.

Taxes are another mechanism by which the total economic system affects the health system. In the last few years, droves of practitioners have incorporated in order to take advantage of a range of tax benefits available to the professional corporation but not to the private practitioner. Tax laws could be used as an inducement for certain type practice situations such as an inner city or group practice—this is hardly farfetched in view of the financial incentives and disincentives Great Britain has used in order to make its system workable. Another area for concern is the occasional grumbling about the tax-exempt status of hospitals and other not-for-profit facilities and organizations. Many of these institutions own considerable real estate and produce revenue from questionably related activities. So far, judicial opinions have tended to favor the tax-exempt institutions in cases such as those concerning medical office buildings. The door has been opened to questions on the tax-exempt status for not-for-profit health care organizations, however, and further challenges should be expected.

The key to effective management in the face of such environmental changes is having a good early warning or scanning system. Theoretically, such a system could cost the equivalent of a talented and expensive front office staff, which is considerably more than most organizations can afford. To a large extent, at the national and regional levels these scanning activities can be carried out by representative organizations, such as the American Hospital Association, the American

Medical Association, or a state hospital association. Trends can be discerned by an organization that has made a commitment to be part of the larger economic and social picture in a region or community. Boards can be most helpful in pinpointing trends likely to affect an organization, but management must want to know what is happening—it must have an appetite for the future. Without this appetite, the organization will eventually find itself with problems that could have been avoided. Illustrative of this situation is one hospital that was located at the edge of the commuter belt of a metropolitan area. Although most members of the community were employed in the local areas, perhaps 30 percent of the work force commuted the 45 miles into the city. A member of the board was the chief executive officer of the largest industry in the community, which employed over 5,000 people. Several years earlier his company had been taken over by a large conglomerate, and the plan was to move the plant to the South within the next few years. The administrator of the hospital never discussed the industry's business with its chief executive officer and had no idea that a move was in the works until it was announced in the local papers. An expansion being considered by the hospital was effectively scrapped or at least put on hold when the information about the impending transfer came to light. While it can be argued that the chief executive officer should have initiated talks with the administrator, it was the administrator who wanted to expand and should have been concerned about the environment. Or, to put it another way, it was the administrator's problem.

STRENGTHS AND WEAKNESSES

The next step in the strategic planning process is perhaps the most difficult in that it requires the organization to identify its strengths and weaknesses. As noted earlier, the identification of strengths is psychologically easier than the identification of weaknesses. It is imperative, however, that those areas where the organization is vulnerable be identified; otherwise, the organization cannot be protected. A framework for considering strengths and weaknesses might be (1) demand for services; (2) capacity for delivering services; (3) competition—present and projected; (4) market position; and (5) cost position.

Demand for Services

A consideration of demand for services could begin with an examination of the usefulness and/or substitutes for the "product" being offered. To an extent, health services are monopoly items, and consumers have little choice but to use health care practitioners and their organizations. However, change that can affect demand does indeed occur in the health care field. For example, in a number of states, optometrists are now allowed to use diagnostic drugs to dilate the pupils, thus resulting in a more effective eye examination. This expansion of the optometrists' scope of licensure has taken place in a heated arena in which ophthalmologists claimed that the dangers inherent in optometrists' using drugs were so great that it should not be allowed. Despite this opposition, 22 states at last count have extended the licensure of optometrists and have in a real sense allowed the consumer to substitute a nonphysician private practitioner for a physician private practitioner.

The past decade has brought other changes. As noted earlier, the legalization of first trimester abortions has resulted in a demand for services that were simply unavailable (legally) before the Supreme Court decisions. Safer and more convenient methods of family planning and changing public attitudes have resulted in a declining birth rate. New technology has given rise to organ transplants and a range of surgery that makes the notion of a "bionic person" not so unrealistic. On a long-run basis, all of this and more must be considered when the health care organization assesses its strengths and weaknesses. For example, is the mix of services being offered what is needed in the community? Does the demographic data in the area suggest that a different mix of services would be more appropriate today? Next year? In five years? Is today's success preventing the consideration of the formula needed to be successful two years from today?

Capacity for Delivering Services

The second area for consideration is the capacity for delivering services—or, to what extent does the present organization have the ability to deliver quality services at a competitive price? This is a function of a variety of factors, including the quality and price of the organization's labor force and its physical facilities. One hospital was extremely competitive because it had an old facility that had been totally depreciated and was in relatively good shape. A new facility at today's prices, however, would have made its cost of services two or three times higher than that of the best teaching hospital in the area.

Competition

For years the notion that health care organizations competed with one another was avoided. Competition for physicians and patients does take place, however, albeit on a professional level and usually in subtle ways. Planners must consider both present and projected competition. In the case of a hospital-based group practice, competition might come from the private practitioners associated with the hospital, physicians practicing in a hospital-owned or hospital-operated office building, the emergency room in the hospital, other group practices in the community, or operating or planned health maintenance organizations.

Market Position and Cost Position

Once the sources of competition have been identified, it is necessary to assess the organization's market position. To what extent can it compete effectively with others offering similar services? Many factors come into play here, such as the organization's image, physical location, quality of facilities, reputation of practitioners, and cost. In the health care field, this last element may or may not be too significant, depending on the nature of the source of payment. If the organization is an ambulatory care program in which there is likely to be a fair degree of self-payment by the patient, cost might be an important element in the total market position. Cost is related to a host of factors, such as efficiency of equipment, cost and productivity of labor, and the quality of the organization's operating systems. In considering cost, the opportunity cost to the patient of utilizing the program or facility should be analyzed, and ways of minimizing those costs should be sought. For example, what can an outstanding diagnostic center located in an out of the way place, such as the Mayo Clinic or the Geisinger Clinic, do to make it easier for a patient to stay there for a few days for diagnostic tests? The Oschner Clinic's solution was building a hotel and restaurant next to its clinic and hospital; this facility could be used by those visiting their suburban New Orleans location for an ambulatory workup or by the families of those hospitalized.

Having worked through this internal and external evaluation, strategic planning now calls for the delineation of alternatives and the selection of the best strategy to meet these stated objectives within the constraints presented. In business schools, a popular case that is used in strategic planning is that of the Head Ski Company. In the late 1950s and early 1960s, the Head Ski Company dominated the U.S. ski market. The company marketed a very small line of high quality merchandise that was essentially the most technically advanced ski in the country—a metal laminated ski invented by Howard Head, the company's founder and chief executive. By the mid-1960s, the company is losing ground to the new, lighter, and more colorful Fiberglas skis arriving from Japan, and within a few years the company has lost its leadership position in this rapidly expanding industry. Head is portrayed as an inventor more concerned with fine-tuning the edges of his skis than making a dollar in the marketplace; the world is portrayed as having an insatiable demand for high technology skis; and the Head Company is portrayed as being committed to only one technology, the metal laminate, and to one color, black. The question posed to the class is: what do you do?

There are many analogues to Head Ski in the health care field, and the following case is presented so that the notions of strategic planning can be applied in a "test situation."

CASE STUDY

Hunterdon Medical Center

For more than 20 years, hospital administrators, trustees, medical staff, and health planners have journeyed to the town of Flemington in west central New Jersey to visit the 200-bed Hunterdon Medical Center. Their attention has been drawn to this institution, located in a semirural community of 75,000 people, not simply because it is a good hospital, but primarily because of the unique health system of 400-square-mile Hunterdon County.

The system consists of a hospital with 35 full-time salaried specialists, 18 residents in family practice, 2 primary care group practices, and 30 family practitioners located in private practice in the 26 municipalities throughout the county. The visitor to Hunterdon sees a closed system where hospital-based physicians serve as specialist consultants to the family practitioner, and family practitioners provide a range of ambulatory and inpatient services and handle almost half of all hospital admissions. In this system, the emergency room is not cluttered with nonurgent problems, patients apparently have access to family-centered comprehensive care, primary care is delivered in the community, and secondary and tertiary care are provided at the hospital. In short, this community is fully involved with its hospital.

Invariably, visitors to Hunterdon Medical Center ask one fundamental question: "How replicable is Hunterdon; that is, can the model of the Hunterdon Medical Center be reproduced elsewhere?" The fast answer is "No," the explanation being that "Hunterdon is unique, it was started in a medical vacuum, and its survival and growth depended on that vacuum. To attempt a transplant where there is not a confluence of community needs, lack of services, and a highly motivated staff would likely be unsuccessful." Despite this seemingly pessimistic appraisal of the replicability of Hunterdon, a study of its complex organization offers significant insights to those interested in hospital-based care. These insights relate to the nature and importance of leadership, community involvement, medical staff organization, and planning.

HISTORY OF HUNTERDON MEDICAL CENTER

In January, 1946, the proposal for a hospital in Hunterdon County was presented to the county's Board of Agriculture. The subject was discussed and debated for the next year, and finally the board asked Dr. E.H.L. Corwin of the New York Academy of Medicine to survey the county's health and hospital needs. Dr. Corwin's comprehensive study, delivered to the board in January, 1948, basically suggested that the county consider building a hospital, but:

To sum up, if Hunterdon County were to build just another hospital, I would be lukewarm to the proposition, but if this hospital is projected in terms of a progressive institution with a university affiliation, a model of its kind, aimed to bring what is best in medicine to the residents of a rural area, and has associated with it an active, full-fledged health center and a good follow-through social service, I would be strongly for it. It should not be difficult for such an institution to secure a good-size endowment. The opportunity is here, and there is unquestionably enough pride and business enterprise in this community to bring this plan for a hospital and health center to successful consummation.

Successfully consummate they did! In March, 1948, incorporation papers were filed, and the Hunterdon Medical Center was launched. A subsequent report by Dr. Corwin in August, 1948, offered the philosophic underpinnings that have guided much of this institution's development:

The hospital as envisioned by the incorporators is not to be a medical hotel or a nursing home, as many hospitals unfortunately are, nor is it to be patterned after the Mayo Clinic or the Lahey Clinic. It is to be a true community hospital which will provide adequate hospital care to the inhabitants of the county, a health protection service and a diagnostic service for the convenience of local physicians. Recognizing that the care of the sick in rural areas, and for that matter in the cities, devolves upon the general practitioner, the Hunterdon Medical Center wishes to provide the physicians in the county utmost opportunities for professional development now and in the future, thus making the highest type of medical service possible.

In other words, it is the intention of the Hunterdon Medical Center to give to the practitioners in the county a firsthand opportunity to participate in the development of the proposed institution and to pave the way for others to continue the work in the community as well-qualified practitioners, abreast of the times not only through secondhand information but from active association with a first-class medical institution. Such an ultimate result is feasible if the hospital from its very inception is dedicated to that ideal and is developing as a teaching unit. It is important to realize that when the hospital becomes, for the time being at least, a part of a collaborative project of a progressive medical school, its organization and its efficiency become the concern and responsibility of the medical school. There are definite practical advantages which accrue from a close association with a university. [Therefore] the Trustees of the prospective medical center have entered into negotiations with the authorities of the New York University-Bellevue Medical Center, and a tentative plan of an alliance has been worked out which would be to the advantage of the hospital and would make it possible for the University Medical Center to fulfill the obligation, recognized by it as well as by some other universities, of extending its influence beyond the teaching of undergraduate medical students. If the plan succeeds, it will result not only in a first-class hospital for the 37,000 people of Hunterdon County, but in a training unit which will set the highest standards for the young people who work and study in it. As a result, the New York University-Bellevue Medical Center, as well as other medical training centers, may be encouraged to establish similar associations elsewhere.

When questioned recently about the importance of this medical-school affiliation for the intellectual health and welfare of the medical center, the president of the Hunterdon Medical Center's Board of Trustees, who has held this position since its founding, stated, "I think the medical school affiliation in the early days was absolutely essential to us." The affiliation allowed the center, in his opinion, to attract a higher caliber of specialist physicians and insured those physicians continued contact with the "mainstream of medical care."

Funding was also a rather important (and, in some quarters, legendary) element in the development of Hunterdon. Of particular interest were the community's financial support of the hospital and the involvement of private foundations in January, 1949, when the project had a bank balance of $240. Eleven months and countless auctions, fairs, theater parties, meetings, and personal solicitations later, more than $900,000 in pledges had been secured from over 70 percent of the county's families—all this in a nonaffluent community without professional fund-raisers.

Finally, one must consider the significance of seed money in the community's quest for medical care. When asked the importance of the several hundred thousand dollars received from the Commonwealth Fund and Kress Foundation in terms of the opening, survival, and success of the Hunterdon Medical Center, the board's president replied:

Absolutely essential. We had just the concept, the vaguest kind of concept, and opened our fund drive. We planned the hospital during the Korean War—until the time we started taking bids, prices soared. We cut almost a million dollars out of the building at the last minute and still the prices came in at about $900,000 more than we had money for. We had promised the community that all the money we had raised would be held in escrow. The only money we spent was Trustees' money. If we couldn't get the job done, we'd give the money back. We had a community council then of about 125 people from all the communities that had been active in fund-raising. We called them together and said,

"Look, if you go broke, the Commonwealth Fund agrees to give us
$250,000 if the community will go in debt for $650,000."
So we called the people together and gave them three options:
1. Give the money back.
2. To forget the University, forget everything, forget Commonwealth
and build a little hospital in the middle of Flemington.
3. Go for broke!
Nobody voted to give the money back. Two said, "The little hospital."
Everybody else said, "Go for broke!"
Had the people chosen otherwise we would have been dead at that point.

On July 3, 1953, the Hunterdon Medical Center opened with 95 beds, 8
full-time physicians, and a staff of 55 employees. Twenty-two years later, it is still
the center of the county's health system and in many respects is a reasonably
accurate reflection of the dreams and aspirations of its planners.

ORGANIZATIONAL ARRANGEMENTS

Since its inception, the basic structure of the 24-member board has not changed,
but the nature of the administrative organization responsible to the board has
evolved from that of a medical director (physician) with a single administrator to
that of a medical director in the top slot with several specialized administrators at
the next level. These five assistant directors are responsible for medical affairs,
administration, finances, data processing, and nursing. Formal coordination of
this six-member management team is handled at a weekly meeting; informal
coordination is carried out continuously.

The board's president, who has an office in the hospital, is involved to an
unusual extent in the functioning of the institution. This close working relationship
between hospital and board has clearly worked at Hunterdon. But one wonders
about the future, when the present board leadership passes on. Will others be able
to provide the same time and dedication to the organization? If not, will the health
and welfare of the institution be jeopardized by that lack of external leadership?

The present medical director is an orthopedist who still practices 25 percent of
his time, serves as both chief executive and chief of staff, and generally coordinates activities with the board. He sees the future of institutional leadership as not
necessarily coming from the founding fathers or first wave of recruits, but perhaps
instead from outside the institution—from physicians in community medicine who
tend to be more interested in health care delivery than in the more narrowly
construed discipline of hospital administration.

Interviews with the assistant directors for administration, nursing, finance, and
data processing suggest that the functions of these people are not significantly

different from those of their counterparts in other community hospitals. The one executive position that clearly differs is that of the assistant director for medical affairs. The functions of this position include the traditional ones as well as those of a medical group manager. For example, the present incumbent deals with professional and nonprofessional staff recruiting, salary levels, and staff evaluation. Most recently, he has developed new methods of remuneration for the full-time staff.

Organization of Clinical Services

All physicians associated with Hunterdon Medical Center practice on a fee-for-service basis, some as hospital-employed physicians and others as community practitioners. Those who are hospital based and physically located at the hospital come from the traditional medical specialties, such as surgery, internal medicine, and ophthalmology. In addition to these specialists, the hospital employs two board-eligible family practitioners who provide patient care and clinical teaching at the Phillips Barber Health Center in Lambertville, 12 miles southwest of Hunterdon. The 30 community physicians—all of whom are board-certified or board-eligible family practitioners and 75 percent of whom were trained at Hunterdon—have offices in a variety of locations throughout the county and generally operate in an individualistic manner.

The structure of the hospital's active medical staff is an important mechanism for linking the hospital physicians and the community practitioners. Medical staff committees are composed of an equal number of full-time hospital-based physicians and community practitioners. An obvious manifestation of both the sharing of responsibility for patients and the mutual respect that generally exists is the observation that the family practitioners admit and care for approximately 50 percent of the hospital's patients. Furthermore, both groups are involved in the family-practice residency program, which has a total of 18 residents (six each in the first, second, and third years). Perhaps most important, both groups seem to view each other as integral to their own professional, financial, and, indeed, intellectual well-being.

The full-time staff is organized into a number of services corresponding generally with those of any other community hospital. These departments carry out the traditional administrative responsibilities; that is, they organize call schedules, plan for growth and development of services, and ensure the delivery of high-quality services. There is, however, one important difference—the director of services is the primary negotiator with the medical director for the salaries of the physicians on his service. This negotiation is directly concerned with the operations of the Professional Service Fund, which is the heart, and perhaps the most controversial aspect, of the financing system for full-time physicians.

The following excerpts from the memorandum of agreement (dated January, 1973), which was signed by the full-time staff, describes this fund:

Professional Service Fund

A. The Professional Service Fund shall consist of:
    1. All funds derived from patient fees and from other professional services rendered by members of the full-time staff with the exception of royalties.
    2. Funds accruing from a division between the Professional Service Fund and the regular operating account of the Medical Center of money received for combined professional-technical services. (In the case of laboratory and X-ray charges, 70 percent to go to operations, 30 percent to PSF. In the case of electrocardiography and electroencephalography, 50 percent each to operations and PSF.)
    3. Such other funds as may specifically be contributed, donated, or granted from time to time in support of education, research, health and other professional activities performed by members of the fulltime staff under the direction of the Medical Director, as authorized by the Board of Trustees.

B. The Professional Service Fund shall be expended by the Board of Trustees of Hunterdon Medical Center for the following purposes:
    1. Salaries of members of the fulltime staff.
    2. Reimbursement to the regular operating account of the Medical Center for the salaries of auxiliary personnel, overhead, administrative services, supplies, maintenance, *et cetera,* required by members of the fulltime staff in the performance of their duties. The amount of the reimbursement shall be determined by the Board of Trustees at the end of each fiscal year on the basis of a cost study conducted by a competent firm of accountants, and after a conference between the Professional Affairs Committee of the Board of Trustees, and Finance Committee of the fulltime staff and the Medical Director. Decisions shall be based on the understanding that income from the professional services provided by members of the fulltime staff shall not be used to cover regular operating expenses of the hospital, nor shall ordinary hospital income be used to subsidize services rendered by members of the fulltime staff.
    3. Retirement program, membership in professional associations, insurance, travel, *et cetera,* as enumerated below.

Since the hospital's inception, the method of paying the physicians has undergone two major changes; and, according to some observers, more are likely. Originally, all physicians received the same salary regardless of specialty or billings, with slight variations based on longevity. In 1965, an incentive plan was introduced that provided the physicians with bonuses based on productivity, teaching, and community service. This system, which had few mechanisms for controlling overhead and an inadequate mechanism for monitoring productivity, resulted in increased overhead charged to the Professional Service Fund.

The newest plan, which is presently in force, provides each department with a prospective budget. This involves a series of negotiations between the department (primarily its director) and the hospital (primarily the medical director) over the objectives, anticipated volumes and expenses, needed resources, and services of the department. These negotiations result in a contract-type agreement between the department and the hospital for services and salaries. The effectiveness of the new plan is yet to be evaluated, but the historical development of this, as well as the previous financial mechanism, demonstrate the need for an organization to respond in an individualized manner to the drives of professionals. Seemingly, the idea of one salary level for all was acceptable at the earlier stages of the Hunterdon Medical Center's development; but, as time passed, physicians simply became more interested in being remunerated in some relation to what they considered their outside earning capacity.

Central to the functioning of both the hospital and the system of health care in the county is the hospital's closed-specialist-staff policy. This policy, incorporated in the bylaws, grants active staff privileges only to physician specialists who are *hospital based.* An eminently well-trained and well-respected specialist or subspecialist actively practicing in the immediate environs of the Hunterdon Medical Center would not, under the present bylaws, be eligible to hospitalize his patients and remain as their attending physician at the hospital. In the past several years, a number of specialists have considered entering private practice in the community, but, learning of the regulations denying them admitting privileges at the hospital, they moved on.

In response to the question "Have there actually been any legal challenges to this closed-staff situation?" the president of the board stated:

> No, nobody has actually taken this to court. We have been threatened by court suit on four or five occasions, but they read our bylaws and they accept the fact that we say this has worked for Hunterdon, and challenge it if you will, this is our position. It has worked for Hunterdon and we think that we are entitled to keep it.

> And the people of Hunterdon have put many millions into this unit and this is what has been working for them, and we're not about to change it. And they back away somehow.

The assistant director for medical affairs added:

> Our legal defense is predicated on our ability to demonstrate that we are meeting the community's demand for care. For example, if a physician approaches us and announces his intention to practice ophthalmology in downtown Flemington on Main Street, we would say, "We have a closed staff, and we are meeting community need in your specialty; therefore, we do not need any additional physicians in your specialty." If, on the other hand, we fail to meet the community's need for service in that specialty, we could be vulnerable to a successful legal action to obtain admitting privileges.

Finally, of fundamental importance to the whole system is the relationship that exists between the full-time and community practitioners, which is one of mutual respect, mutual concern, and, indeed, admiration for one another's work. While this may be a result of a close relationship developed with the full-time staff during the community practitioners' training period (75 percent of the county's family practitioners are trained at Hunterdon), it is also no doubt related to the relatively clear delineation of professional authority and responsibility for patient care. In general, the family practitioners handle ambulatory and inpatient primary care, leaving ambulatory and inpatient secondary care for the hospital-based specialists. However, there are family doctors who do manage patients on services that are traditionally considered secondary and tertiary in nature. For example, a number of the family doctors admit coronary patients to the intensive care unit and manage them without a specialty consultation, yet the family doctor is not operating independently, for his patient is constantly surrounded by students, house staff, and full-time members.

Ambulatory Care Organization

Ambulatory care is provided in the family practitioners' offices throughout the county, the specialists' offices at the hospital, the hospital emergency room, the Riverfield Medical Group P.A. in Clinton, the Delaware Valley Family Health Center in Milford, and the Phillips Barber Family Health Center in Lambertville. The last center is operated by the hospital as a primary care facility and is staffed by hospital-employed family practitioners.

Under optimal conditions, each patient would have as his first line of contact a family practitioner who, in addition to providing primary care, would be responsible for coordinating secondary and tertiary care activities. A description of this mechanism in practice appeared in the November, 1968, issue of *Hospital Physician,* in which the case of a carpenter whose eye had been hit by a flying nail is discussed by a Hunterdon County family practitioner:

As soon as I saw that the eye was severely damaged—more seriously than I could handle—I called Dr. J.W., one of the two ophthalmologists at the Medical Center. He said, "Send him in" and two hours later he called me back to say the nail had pierced the cornea and that the man would be hospitalized for three or four days. After this man is discharged, Dr. J.W. will follow him for his eye problem, and then send him back to me. I will bill the patient for an office visit and I will see him in the hospital because I feel a personal obligation to see that he's well cared for. But I won't bill for these visits. They're just courtesy calls.

With few exceptions, family practitioners are in solo practice and carry on in an independent manner, choosing their own location, billing their patients separately, keeping their own style of medical records, and arranging their own office hours, vacations, coverage, and patient load. In general, this seems to work well: several studies and personal observations indicate that most people have a sense of being tied into the system. A clear manifestation of the system's effectiveness is the low utilization of the Hunterdon Medical Center's emergency room for primary care (an estimated 15-30 percent of the patient visits).

A recent development in family practice is the hospital's sponsorship of primary care group practice in two separate ways. This sponsorship was necessitated by the fact that practitioners were simply not moving to Hunterdon County, where medical care was needed.

The first approach is that of the Phillips Barber Family Health Center. This strikingly attractive facility of 5,000 square feet, built by bequests from the Phillips Barber Foundation, provides primary health care for approximately 7,000 people, and serves as a model unit for the medical center's family practice residency program, as required by the American Medical Association's Council on Medical Education in its "Essentials of Approved Residencies." The facility is staffed by two full-time hospital-employed family practitioners and four full-time-equivalent residents. There are daily record reviews, a continual informal audit system, and a sophisticated system of tracking morbidity of ambulatory patients.

The center's prime mission is to provide good, family-centered, accessible primary care. Toward those ends, medical records are kept on a family basis; the center is open from 8:30 a.m. to 5:00 p.m., weekends, Monday and Thursday evenings, and Saturday mornings from 8:30 a.m. to 11:30 a.m.; and physicians are on call and make house calls. A relatively self-sufficient operation, the center conducts basic laboratory work-ups, is involved in community health education, and contracts with a nonprofit transportation service (Progress on Wheels) for patients unable to get there themselves. The gross billings of the Phillips Barber Center in 1973 were $200,000, and the operating loss was calculated at $34,000 (a figure equal to the amount budgeted for indirect Hunterdon Medical Center expenses, that is, computers and administration).

The second approach to sponsorship of primary care group practice taken by the Hunterdon Medical Center can be seen at the Riverfield Medical Group, P.A., in Clinton. Here two physicians have leased the hospital's practice building. The *quid pro quo* of this arrangement is that the medical group pays rent plus its own utilities, housekeeping, and staffing costs, and the practice serves as a teaching unit for the Hunterdon Medical Center's residency program in family practice. The hospital, for its part, built the $280,000 building on land it was given and maintains the facility. The rental fee is set at a low level to offset the teaching provided by the physicians. Primary care services, medical records, and auxiliary services are handled in Clinton similarly to those at the Phillips Barber Center, with one major difference—the Clinton physicians are family practitioners who are not hospital-employed.

The county's ambulatory care specialists are based at the Hunterdon Medical Center. Thirty-five full-time specialists provide a full range of services in the diagnostic center of the hospital, which is open eight hours a day, five days a week. Each specialty service organizes its own activities, such as appointment systems and coverage. Although no formal mechanisms exist to control patient volume, an informal mechanism operates through discouragement of self-referrals and the general lack of primary care capability at the hospital. In addition, the physicians are generally recruited to the staff for their specialty expertise, not for their general medical care abilities. Thus, a cardiologist would be expected to function mainly in his specialist capacity.

New patients arriving at the hospital for ambulatory care are not required to have their complete histories taken and to undergo physical examinations; nor are specialty- or subspecialty-referred patients required to have any type of standard examinations. It is thus not only possible but probable that, despite the system's closed nature, patients receive episodic and fragmented specialty care. Records are centralized, and inpatient and hospital-based ambulatory service records are stored together on opposite sides of the same folder. However, when medical records are reviewed, the audit focuses on the inpatient side.

How is quality maintained in ambulatory care? The answer is primarily related to the hospital's commitment to medical education. As a medical-school-affiliated teaching institution, the hospital considers all its patients teaching patients and therefore provides them care—whether by a resident, specialist, or family practitioner—that is constantly under formal and informal review.

This overriding commitment also results in the recruitment and selection of well-trained and highly motivated physicians. Finally, there are a host of intra and extramural scientific and educational meetings with which professional staff are involved. For example, all full-time staff physicians are on the clinical faculty of Rutgers Medical School, where many of them spend a day each week. Locally, there are medical staff meetings on the second Tuesday of every month (including educational sessions) and regular scientific meetings every Saturday morning, but these are reported to be sparsely attended.

By almost any standard, the Hunterdon Medical Center is an eminently successful organization. Prior to its inception, the people in Hunterdon County had few health care resources. Today, they have a modern health system that provides a wide range of services in a high quality, comprehensive, accessible, and available manner.

CASE ANALYSIS

Is the Hunterdon Medical Center a "success"? The issue of success can involve a variety of criteria, e.g., the financial stability of the organization, its growth, and its community support. On virtually any criterion, except perhaps physician satisfaction, the Medical Center has been successful. Even on this criterion, it appears that problems have been limited until recently.

A second question that should be asked is, How successful is the center likely to be in the future? In order to answer this question those factors that led to its success in the first instance must be considered. Paramount among these factors was a post-World War II boom in the economy that brought industry, housing, and money to Hunterdon County. Second, there was a medical vacuum in the county prior to the center's establishment, and even those general practitioners already located there had no readily accessible inpatient facility. The geographical isolation of the county also worked to the benefit of the Medical Center in that it provided an almost natural catchment area for patients. A fourth factor was the excitement generated in the community over having its own hospital and the spirit of those people involved at the inception of what was viewed as a major innovation. Other factors that no doubt contributed to the success of the Medical Center were the affiliation with a medical school, professional interest in rural medicine, the attractiveness of rural Hunterdon County as a place to live and work, the dynamic medical and board leadership in the new hospital, the lack of competition, the attractiveness of physical facilities and potential for expansion, and the unique organizational set-up with family practitioners working in the community and with the salaried hospital-based specialists.

Now that the reasons for current success have been analyzed, what is needed for success in the future and how have things changed since the opening of the Medical Center? The most obvious change has been in the size and nature of the community, which has had a 100 percent growth in population. This growth is in large part related to the fact that the county has become a bedroom community for New York City and Philadelphia commuters. Because two recently opened interstate highways transect the county, this type of growth will probably continue. All of this suggests that the county may become more suburban in nature and that attitudes toward use of family practitioners may shift. For example, will the new residents want to receive their primary care from a family practitioner or internist, since the latter pattern is more prevalent in the cities?

A second important change since the center's inception is that community support has decreased significantly. Only several hundred thousand dollars per year are now collected by the annual fund drive, and that money is from a small number of contributors. In line with the earlier discussion of motivation, it might be hypothesized that the Medical Center is no longer a "motivation" factor in the community but rather a "hygiene" factor. Thus, as the Medical Center goes out to compete (in whatever arena), it cannot expect the same level of enthusiastic support it enjoyed in the past.

A final and crucial point is that, as the Medical Center has moved through its puberty and adolescence into adulthood, so has the rest of the nation in terms of trying to organize and control the health system. In the late 1940s when the Center was being conceived and in the 1950s when it was establishing itself, much of what was happening happened in a vacuum. Health planning and regulation were in their infancy, and the role of the federal government in the financing and direction of hospitals was relatively minimal. Now Hunterdon must consider what other institutions in the area are doing or want to do, and this introduces an element of competition with other institutions and programs that simply did not exist 20 years ago.

In fact, subsequent to the preparation of this case, competitive and regulatory developments in New Jersey did create problems for the Medical Center. For example, one crucial issue stemmed from the high daily costs and short length of stay for hospitalized patients, payment for which was in part disallowed by the state since the costs were out of range with those of other similar-sized hospitals. For Hunterdon, the net result was a dangerous deficit. A time- and money-consuming appeal that was resolved unsatisfactorily (from the hospital's perspective) pointed out that Hunterdon was a victim of its own success. The staff attempted to keep patients out of the hospital—thus, when they were hospitalized, the hospitalization tended to be more intensive. The state's approach of looking simply at aggregated data for length of stay clearly worked to the hospital's detriment.

The next important question is, What other threats would seem to exist? Competition poses a real threat to the Medical Center because it is so firmly based on the concept of cooperation between a full-time specialist staff and community-based family practitioners. A group of physicians from the Medical Center could leave the full-time practice of the institution, set up practice across the street, and demand admitting privileges into the Medical Center. While in the past the institution has been able to resist these attempts to break into its closed staff, there are legal and political reasons to believe that such attempts could not be blocked if a serious court challenge were undertaken.

A second and related problem is the institution's need to expand and capture different population groups for primary care in order to provide the conduit for secondary care and hospitalizations that are the lifeblood of the Medical Center. Indeed, the more successful the entire system is at keeping patients out of the hospital, the more it is necessary for the hospital to expand its population base in order to maintain the services and staff of the hospital. One response to these problems has been the establishment of two satellite clinics and the planning of a third. Since each of these clinics is set up on a different management model and has a different relationship with the Medical Center, the authority and responsibility of the Medical Center vis-à-vis these new programs must be clarified.

In many respects, all of these problems come together in one question. Where will the next generation of leadership come from? A review of this case shows that the top management staff of this institution is somewhat different from that of most facilities in that the unsalaried president of the board de facto functions as the (almost) full-time chief executive officer of the Medical Center. He appears to be an extremely strong person surrounded by a relatively weak board and administration. While this type of leadership may have been necessary to develop Hunterdon to its present point, the need for new blood has apparently not been addressed. There is no management team ready to take over, and it appears that the medical staff has not developed to a point where it can meet future challenges. For the past few years, the physicians on the staff have expended much of their energy on conflicts over finances, and these conflicts have prevented them from organizing themselves to challenge the leadership. Could a threat from them topple the leadership? If so, what are the implications for the future of the Medical Center?

A list of external factors that are most likely to affect the Medical Center would certainly include the opening of the county to suburbanization by the interstate highways and the increased costs of energy, inflation, and wages. As noted earlier, federal and state regulations will be prominent in Hunterdon's future, as will the effects of population growth, the higher educational level of the new residents, and the development of the New Jersey College of Medicine and Surgery. Because of its two campuses and its interest in primary care, this medical school could potentially have an important impact on the developments in Hunterdon.

By means of the model utilized for considering the strengths and weaknesses, each of the components of the Medical Center can be examined separately: first, the personal component—the consumers; second, the professional component, which is composed of the providers; and, finally, the organizational component of the Medical Center.

In terms of strength, the consumers present a unique case for a nonprepaid situation; they have effectively enrolled in the Medical Center. They appear to view it as their Medical Center and tend to be loyal to it. Few Hunterdon County residents obtain their medical care out of the county or area. In many senses then, the Medical Center has a defined population base and a loyal one at that. Such definition and loyalty allow plans to be made on the basis of more reliable data than are normally encountered.

From a provider perspective, Hunterdon has well-trained specialists and family practitioners who are well located throughout the community and appear, through their medical school affiliations, to be quality oriented.

In terms of the organization, there are a number of strengths. First, unlike most hospitals, this organization has an ideology that to some extent focuses its efforts. Its strong president provides important leadership, which has resulted in a positive reputation nationally and good relationships locally. The hospital has a good physical facility; therefore, the myriad operational problems that can become debilitating are unlikely in the foreseeable future. Finally, the hospital is a central part of the total health system. This has both conceptual value and practical importance. For example, because of its centrality, the hospital is the receiver of almost all secondary referrals and inpatients.

The Medical Center has several weaknesses. As noted earlier, the consumers are changing, their tastes are changing, and they may not want to use the system as it was constructed and is intended to be used. Within the traditional Hunterdon community, the hospital has certainly lost much of its glamour—it is not disliked, but it has become "institutionalized." Provider weaknesses include three very serious issues. First, there is a conflict over money. Who shall get how much and under what circumstances? Part of this conflict has to do with who shall control the disbursement of these funds. A second weakness is the apparent ideological conflict among members of the medical staff and between some members of the medical staff and the president over the "system." A manifestation of this conflict was the health maintenance organization (HMO) feasibility study that was considered several years earlier. Some members of the medical staff were strongly in favor of developing an HMO and viewed it as a natural extension of the activities and concerns of Hunterdon, while others considered it totally inappropriate. This is an interesting example of how the same system and institution can be considered liberal by one group and conservative by another group. To some, Hunterdon is a rather liberal, perhaps radical, experiment in American medical care in that it essentially develops the British National Health System without the financing mechanism. To others, it is quite conservative in that it organizes the providers and institutions into a relationship that maximizes each physician's professional situation and effectively forces the consumer into an ideal professional model. A final problem concerning providers, which was only becoming apparent as this case was prepared, involves the low productivity of the physicians.

From an organizational standpoint, some of those factors identified as strengths are also weaknesses; they are indeed two-edged swords. For example, the ideology can be viewed as positive, but it is also a hindrance to the development of the Medical Center. Perhaps the ideology is too rigid on competition—competition might be healthy for those on staff and might also provide a safety valve for those on staff who want an opportunity to go into private practice. Other weaknesses include the problem of one-person dominance—in this case, the board president—and its related weak board and poor medical staff leadership. What happens if the president drops out for any reason?

A different sort of weakness has to do with the development of the satellites, which commits the resources of the institution to towns that should have been able to attract physicians without such a special commitment. What can be said about a system that trains family practitioners who are unwilling to practice 10 or 15 miles away from the Medical Center in communities where there is a clear need and where good incomes are practically guaranteed?

A related weakness is "nepotism" in that 75 percent of the family practitioners in Hunterdon County were trained at the Medical Center. This may create problems in terms of development, since almost everyone has gone through the same socialization process. In addition, it is unlikely that physicians will have the experience or desire to challenge future developments in the system in which they were trained. Finally, the system has no long-term care component; thus, the ideology of providing comprehensive care is sorely lacking in what is likely to be a critical need area in the future.

At the final stage of analyzing this case from the strategic planning perspective, the question to be considered is, What strategic planning should be going on? First, the institution should continue developing effective programs to enroll the population. The satellite program is one step in the right direction because it allows primary care to be given in the community while secondary and inpatient care is delivered in the hospital. Part of this strategy of enrolling the population can involve health education; the hospital has already been actively engaged in health education through a variety of community-based programs in its search for new ways to identify with the community.

A second component in the hospital's strategic planning might be professional development of the medical staff, administration, and board. Basically, the institution must prepare the staff for a new generation of leadership. Otherwise, when the change comes, it may be extremely disruptive.

Finally, the organization must develop its relationship with other organizations, in particular the nearby medical school in New Jersey. Quite clearly, Hunterdon does not want to be just another small community hospital—rather, it wishes to be a model, something special. It must then begin to reestablish those relationships that make it something special and find staff who consider it something other than a high quality small community hospital. To some extent, the leadership and old guard retain traces of the old ideology of excellence and public service; unfortunately, much of that "spirit" has been lost in latter day cynicism and translation. It must be recaptured in a variety of positive ways if the hospital is to avoid both organizational banality and chaos.

Postscript

Chaos did come. It came despite excellent and expensive consulting reports by some of the best people in the field. In less than 18 months the hospital was sued by its own medical staff, and the president and medical director resigned. A new president, a nationally prominent physician-administrator, was hired, but he resigned after less than a year. A new (and first) nonphysician director was recruited. The hospital lost considerable money because of New Jersey reimbursement regulations, and somewhat bitter articles appeared in various journals and newspapers predicting the imminent demise of the Hunterdon system. However, a new reimbursement scheme being tested by New Jersey and able administration suggest that Hunterdon will continue as a viable institution. What will happen with the system in the future remains to be seen—but, from the perspective of the former president presented in the *New England Journal of Medicine,* "Camelot is dead."

CASE STUDY

P. LeRoy Farley Hospital Case

The P. LeRoy Farley Hospital is a not-for-profit corporation incorporated on June 30, 1947, as a voluntary, not-for-profit, nonsectarian community hospital. The original 40-bed acute care hospital (the Arden Pavilion) was completed in January, 1951, at its present site in Davis, New York—a suburb approximately 35 miles north of the George Washington Bridge. Thirty-eight beds were added to the Arden Pavilion in 1958. A third construction program was completed in 1974 with the opening of a 200-bed facility (the Columbia Pavilion) on a 30-acre site approximately 2.5 miles from the 4-acre Arden Pavilion site.

The pavilions operate together as a 278-bed acute care general hospital that provides a full range of services, including 190 medical-surgical, 16 pediatric, 32 obstetrical, and 18 intensive and coronary care beds. The institution is fully accredited and is an active member of various professional organizations.

The institution is governed by an 18-member self-perpetuating board of trustees who serve for terms of one, two, or three years and may serve for more than one term. Current officers and members and their business affiliations are as follows:

Albert J. Smedley (President)	Regional Vice President Great National Life Assurance Co.
John V. Clancy (First Vice President)	Deputy Provost Columbia University
Robert Buffalo, M.D. (Second Vice President)	Physician
Mrs. J.J. Clarabell (Third Vice President)	Homemaker
Mrs. Frank Kukla (Secretary)	Homemaker
Thomas Stickyfinger (Treasurer)	Manager, Labor Relations Federal National Banks
Mrs. Winnie Pooh	Advertising Manager *Better Homes & Apartments*
Humphrey Dumpty	President Davis Realty Company
John Sprat	President Sprat Food Centres, Ltd.
O.M. McDonald	Retired Farmer
Benjamin Casey, M.D.	Physician
Hon. Phineas T. Bluster	Congressman, 14th C.D., New York
Redmond R. Rose	President Davis Oldsmobile
Peter A. Rabbit	Editor American Dictionary Co.
Mrs. George Porgi	Homemaker

Mrs. LaMont Hubbard	Homemaker
Rev. H.O. Lee	Minister First Church of Davis
R.H. Mace	Manager Sears, Roebuck and Co.

The administrative staff of the hospital is headed by Pierre LaVantz, who has been director since December, 1973. Prior to being named director, he had been assistant director since 1963. Mr. LaVantz received a B.A. in Biology from New York University and a M.S. in Hospital Administration from Columbia.

Mr. Rollo Kaiser, assistant director, joined the institution in 1972 after holding several other positions in the New York metropolitan area. He has a B.S. from California State College at Fresno and a M.H.A. from the University of Michigan. The deputy assistant administrator is Mr. Phil Bagel, a 1978 graduate of the Yale School of Public Health program in hospital administration.

A total of 212 physicians and dentists, including 72 active, 47 courtesy, 46 consulting, 20 dental, 19 associate, and 8 provisional members, serve on the institution's medical and dental staff. One hundred one members are board-certified in their particular specialties. The average age of the medical and dental staff is 46 years. The medical and dental staff is organized into 13 major departments: anesthesiology, dentistry, family medicine, internal medicine, obstetrics and gynecology, surgery, ophthalmology, orthopedics, pathology, radiology, pediatrics, urology, and emergency room. Specific services offered by the institution include formal, organized clinics in cardiology, medical, obstetrics and gynecology, surgery, and orthopedics. The institution has a respiratory therapy department, which is headed by a registered and certified technician assisted by six certified technicians.

A full-time director of Development responsible for fund-raising activities was employed by the institution in 1977. The institution reports that $632,000 has been raised by this department in its first 33 months of operation.

The Women's Auxiliary of the institution was organized in 1949. Nine active chapters from communities in the institution's service area have maintained on-going fund-raising programs and have raised approximately $750,000 since their inception. The volunteer program of the Women's Auxiliary, which includes Pink Ladies and Candy Stripers, trains and provides volunteers for service throughout the institution. An average of 450 volunteers per month worked an average of 6,820 hours per month, totaling 81,848 volunteer hours in 1979.

The Men's Corps at the institution was organized in 1976 and includes 75 members who work as volunteers in various departments. An average of 40 men per month worked an average of 630 hours per month, recording 7,388 volunteer hours in 1979.

Table 12-1 Percentage Breakdown of Patient Days by Payer Type for 1979

Blue Cross	41%
Medicare	27%
Medicaid	2%
Commercial insurance and self-paying	30%
	100%

A major portion of the institution's revenues are received from third party payers on a cost reimbursement basis. Table 12-1, as reported by the institution, is a percentage breakdown of patient days by payer type for the fiscal year ended December 31, 1979.

Discussion Question

1. A consultant has been approached by Dr. Casey and asked to assist in the selection of a firm to do a financial feasibility study for a new unified facility at the Columbia Pavilion site. Casey is concerned that the board does not really know what is going on, and he feels that LaVantz is purposely keeping everyone in the dark. Casey says there is a lack of trust among the board members and between the board and administration. In addition, the community is changing. What steps should be taken in developing a strategic plan for the organization?

NOTES

1. G.A. Steiner, *Top Management Planning* (Toronto: Collier-MacMillian, 1969), pp. 21-27.
2. M. Crichton, *Five Patients* (New York: Knopf, 1970), pp. 115-154.

Solution to the Health Facilities Location Problem

THE MATHEMATICAL RISK MODEL

Let I be the set $\{1, 2, \ldots, m\}$, representing m different medical services and let $J(i)$, i in I be the set $\{1, 2, \ldots, n_i\}$ of people seeking service i in I.

We assume that a coordinate system has been conveniently established. The natural Euclidean norm is appropriate for this problem. Then let

$\overline{X}_{i,j}$ = the X coordinate of the jth known patient seeking the ith medical service, with i in I and j in $J(i)$.

$\overline{Y}_{i,j}$ = the Y coordinate of the jth known patient seeking the ith medical service, with i in I and j in $J(i)$.

X_i = the X coordinate of the ith medical service, with i in I. X_i is a decision variable.

Y_i = the Y coordinate of the ith medical service, with i in I. Y_i is a decision variable.

r_{ij} = a random variable representing the amount of medical service i required by patient j, with i in I and j in $J(i)$. Let $\mu_{r_{ij}}$ and $\sigma_{r_{ij}}$ stand for the mean and standard deviation of r_{ij}, respectively.

W_{ij} = the amount of medical service i delivered to patient j, with i in I and j in $J(i)$. W_{ij} is a decision variable.

β_{ij} = the known unit cost in dollars per mile per medical service i paid by patient j, with i in I and j in $J(i)$.

It is obvious that the Euclidean distance D_{ij}, traveled by patient j to the unknown location of the ith medical service is given by

$$D_{ij} = [(\overline{X}_{ij} - X_i)^2 + (\overline{Y}_{ij} - Y_i)^2]^{1/2} \qquad (1)$$

for all i in I and all j in $J(i)$.

We will assume that for a fixed service i, i in I, the sequence of random variables $r_{i1}, r_{i2}, \ldots, r_{in_i}$ is independent and identically distributed. We furthermore assume that each random variable r_{ij} is normally distributed with mean $\mu_{r_{ij}}$ and standard deviation $\sigma_{r_{ij}}$.

The risk model to locate the ith facility can then be stated as

$$\text{Min } \ C_i = \sum_{j=1}^{n_i} \beta_{ij} W_{ij} D_{ij} \tag{2}$$

$$\text{st} \quad P[W_{ij} \geq r_{ij}] \geq \alpha_{ij}, \qquad j = 1, \ldots, n_i \tag{3}$$

$$W_{ij} \geq 0, \quad X_i \geq 0, \quad Y_i \geq 0, \qquad j = 1, \ldots, n_i \tag{4}$$

where D_{ij} is given in (1), and $0 \leq \alpha_{ij} \leq 1$ for all i in I and j in $J(i)$. In this formulation P stands for probability and (3) merely says that the probability that the amount of the ith medical service delivered to the jth patient will exceed its required service, must be at least as great as α_{ij}.

The units of the objective function given in (2) are obviously seen to be in dollars. The mathematical model to locate the ith medical facility and the total amount of service delivered at the ith facility as stated in (2), (3), and (4) is a Chance-Constrained Programming Problem.[1]

Before transforming the stochastic formulation to a deterministic one, where algorithms for its solution are in abundance, some commentaries are appropriate.

The values of the α_{ij} to be employed must be attained as additional data from the administration of the ith medical service. The selection of minimum probability levels by the ith medical facility should be based on a balancing of two different "costs." On the one hand, there is the cost of violating a constraint, that is, of not delivering the minimum requirements to a patient. These "costs" must be determined outside the model. In general, the higher the level of α_{ij} selected, the lower the expected level of these costs. On the other hand, there are the costs measured in terms of the objective functions of the model that increase as the probability levels increase, since the problem then becomes more severely constrained. The latter cost can be estimated using parametric programming. It has been suggested that both costs should be captured in the objective functions by including a specific cost associated with the probability with which a constraint will be violated. In short, it has been suggested that the determination of levels for the α_{ij} is properly a part of the optimizing model. This technique requires a means of weighting the cost given by (2) and the other costs associated with the selection of the α_{ij}. The weightings must be determined through the use of a utility function for the ith medical service administration, or we must be satisfied with the determination of efficient points.

If we let $\omega(\alpha_{ij})$ be the "cost" associated with the violation of the jth constraint for the ith medical service, then we are assuming the ith medical service's utility function can be written as

$$U_i[C_i, \omega(\alpha_{i1}), \omega(\alpha_{i2}), \ldots, \omega(\alpha_{in_i})].$$

If we fix each α_{ij} and minimize C_i, we have found one point on the efficiency frontier for the ith medical service. The final choice of a point on the frontier as the *best* for the ith medical service requires complete knowledge of the utility function.[2]

The costs associated with not meeting a patient's minimum requirement will undoubtedly be difficult for the ith medical service administration to measure.* Instead, the ith medical service is more likely to be concerned with some estimate of the frequency with which a patient's requirement will *not* be met, even though it may not be able to convert the frequency directly into cost estimates. In other words, the ith medical service administrator may not be able to estimate the costs of not satisfying the requirements of a particular patient. However, he may have some subjective feelings about how often, on the average, he can disappoint each patient without dire consequences. In short, the α_{ij} parameters used in the relation (3) may be taken to be the subjective estimates of this critical quality of service. The discussion of the dual variables, to follow, offers means of measuring the influence of changes in the α_{ij} estimates on the minimum attainable expected costs.

Let us next transform the chance-constrained programming model ([2], [3], [4]) for the ith medical service into a deterministic nonlinear programming problem subject to linear constraints.

It follows that

$$P[W_{ij} \geq r_{ij}] = P[(W_{ij} - \mu_{r_{ij}})/\sigma_{r_{ij}} \geq (r_{ij} - \mu_{r_{ij}})/\sigma_{r_{ij}}] \geq \alpha_{ij} \qquad (5)$$

The parameters $\mu_{r_{ij}}$ and $\sigma_{r_{ij}}$ are assumed to be estimated from past experience. The terms on the right hand side of each of the bracketed inequalities are standardized random variables with zero means and unitary standard deviations. It is their distribution that is tabulated and known. For example if r_{ij} is normal then $(r_{ij} - \mu_{r_{ij}})/\sigma_{r_{ij}}$ is $N(0,1)$.

If we let $G_{\alpha_{ij}}$ be the abscissa associated with the left tail of the standard distribution function for probability level α_{ij}, as illustrated in Figure 1, then

$$P(W_{ij} \geq r_{ij}) \geq \alpha_{ij} = P\left(\frac{W_{ij} - \mu_{r_{ij}}}{\sigma_{r_{ij}}} \geq \frac{r_{ij} - \mu_{r_{ij}}}{\sigma_{r_{ij}}}\right) \geq \alpha_{ij}.$$

---

* Some work has been done to determine those costs in the framework of industrial supply and distribution systems.[3,4]

Figure 1 Standard Distribution Function for Probability Level α_{ij}

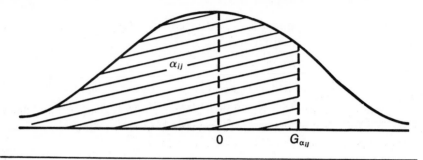

Thus,

$$P\left(G_{\alpha_{ij}} \geq \frac{r_{ij} - \mu_{r_{ij}}}{\sigma_{r_{ij}}}\right) = \alpha_{ij} \Rightarrow \frac{W_{ij} - \mu_{r_{ij}}}{\sigma_{r_{ij}}} \geq G_{\alpha_{ij}}.$$

Finally,

$$W_{ij} \geq G_{\alpha_{ij}} \sigma_{r_{ij}} + \mu_{r_{ij}}.$$

We can thus conclude that

$$P(W_{ij} \geq r_{ij}) \geq \alpha_{ij} \qquad \text{if and only if}$$

$$W_{ij} \geq G_{\alpha_{ij}} \sigma_{r_{ij}} + \mu_{r_{ij}} \qquad \text{for all } i \text{ in } I, \ j \text{ in } J(i).$$

Then the location problem can be written in its deterministic format as

$$\text{Min } C_i = \sum_{j=1}^{n_i} \beta_{ij} W_{ij} D_{ij} \tag{2}$$

$$\text{st} \quad W_{ij} \geq G_{\alpha_{ij}} \sigma_{r_{ij}} + \mu_{r_{ij}}, \qquad j = 1, \ldots, n_i \tag{6}$$

$$W_{ij} \geq 0, \ X_i \geq 0, \ Y_i \geq 0$$

where D_{ij} is given in (1). The constraints (6) are linear in the decision variable because they do not serve as multipliers of the random variable r_{ij}. This is not generally the case in chance-constrained programming.

Since C_i ($C_i \geq 0$) is linear in W_{ij} with $\dfrac{\partial C_i}{\partial W_{ij}} > 0$, it is clear that W_{ij} must be as small as possible; thus (6) reduces to

$$W_{ij} = G_{\alpha_{ij}} \sigma_{r_{ij}} + \mu_{r_{ij}}, \qquad j = 1, \ldots, n_i. \tag{7}$$

Then the location problem reduces to

$$\text{Min } C_i = \sum_{j=1}^{n_i} \beta_{ij}(G_{\alpha_{ij}}\sigma_{r_{ij}} + \mu_{ij})D_{ij} \tag{8}$$

$$\text{st} \quad X_i \geqslant 0, \ Y_i \geqslant 0$$

where D_{ij} is defined in (1).

It has been shown[5,6] that the objective function (8) is convex; thus, there exists a single global minimum for C_i and no additional local minima.

Algorithms to solve (8) will be discussed in the next section.

The solution of (7) and (8) will yield for each medical service i, i in I, a vector

$$(\overline{W}_i, X_i, Y_i) \tag{9}$$

where

$$\overline{W}_i = \sum_{j=1}^{n_i} W_{ij}. \tag{10}$$

The vector (9) will determine the exact location and the total amount of medical services of type i to be delivered. If we follow this procedure m times, we will compute a similar vector for each one of the m different medical services. In general, the mathematical model will suggest m different locations. However, the construction of m different health facilities will incur multiple sets of fixed charges, and thus a unique location containing all m medical services is desirable. This is in fact an easy task. If we let

X_i = the X known coordinate of the ith medical service

Y_i = the Y known coordinate of the ith medical service

$\overline{W}_i$ = the known total amount of service to be delivered at the ith medical facility

γ_i = a known unit cost in dollars per mile per service $i*$

X = the X coordinate of the unique location, X being a decision variable

Y = the Y coordinate of the unique facility, Y being a decision variable,

then the optimal coordinates X and Y are computed from

---

* In this paper $\gamma_i = \dfrac{1}{m}\displaystyle\sum_{i=1}^{m} \beta_{ij}$, for all i in I.

$$\text{Min } \sum_{i=1}^{m} \gamma_i \overline{W}_i D_i \qquad (11)$$

$$\text{st } X \geq 0, \ Y \geq 0 \qquad (12)$$

where
$$D_i = [(X_i - X)^2 + (Y_i - Y)^2]^{1/2}. \qquad (13)$$

It has been shown that (11) is also a convex function,[5,6] and thus there is a unique global minimum.

THE SOLUTION ALGORITHM

Solution techniques to solve (8) or (11) are in abundance. Among others, there are iterative techniques such as Newton's approximation method,[7] steepest descent method,[8,9] various random methods,[10,11,12] branch and bound,[13,14,15] as well as others.[16,17,18,19,20] How rapidly these methods do converge depends on the choice of an initial trial location. The solution given by the center of gravity method is considered to be an efficient starting solution.[6,16,21]

In particular, the algorithm used in this paper is due to Cooper.[12] After setting the dual formulation to (8), Cooper obtains the following recursive equations:

At iteration $k + 1$ ($k \geq 0$ and integer)

$$X_i^{k+1} = \frac{\displaystyle\sum_{j=1}^{n_i} \frac{\beta_{ij} W_{ij} \overline{X}_{ij}}{D_{ij}^k}}{\displaystyle\sum_{j=1}^{n_i} \frac{\beta_{ij} W_{ij}}{D_{ij}^k}} \qquad i = 1, \ldots, m$$

and

$$Y_i^{k+1} = \frac{\displaystyle\sum_{j=1}^{n_i} \frac{\beta_{ij} W_{ij} \overline{Y}_{ij}}{D_{ij}^k}}{\displaystyle\sum_{j=1}^{n_i} \frac{\beta_{ij} W_{ij}}{D_{ij}^k}} \qquad i = 1, \ldots, m$$

where
$$D_{ij}^k = [(X_{ij} - X_i^k)^2 + (Y_{ij} - Y_i^k)^2]^{1/2},$$

$$i = 1, \ldots, m; \qquad j = 1, \ldots, n_i,$$

$$W_{ij} = G_{\alpha_{ij}} \sigma_{r_{ij}} + \mu_{r_{ij}}, \qquad i = 1, \ldots, m; \qquad j = 1, \ldots, n_i,$$

and the initial values X_i^0 and Y_i^0 are chosen from

$$X_i^0 = \frac{\sum\limits_{j=1}^{n_i} \beta_{ij} W_{ij} \overline{X}_{ij}}{\sum\limits_{j=1}^{n_i} \beta_{ij} W_{ij}} \qquad i = 1, \ldots, m$$

$$Y_i^0 = \frac{\sum\limits_{j=1}^{n_i} \beta_{ij} W_{ij} \overline{Y}_{ij}}{\sum\limits_{j=1}^{n_i} \beta_{ij} W_{ij}}$$

The algorithm stops when for a given number $\epsilon_i > 0$,

$$|X_i^{k+1} - X_i^k| < \epsilon_i$$

and   for $i = 1, \ldots, m$.

$$|Y_i^{k+1} - Y_i^k| < \epsilon_i$$

In a similar way, the iterative procedure to solve (11) is as follows. At iteration $k + 1$, ($k \geqslant 0$ and integer)

$$X^{k+1} = \frac{\sum\limits_{i=1}^{m} \frac{\gamma_i \overline{W}_i X_i}{D_i^k}}{\sum\limits_{j=1}^{m} \frac{\gamma_i \overline{W}_i}{D_i^k}}$$

$$Y^{k+1} = \frac{\sum\limits_{i=1}^{m} \frac{\gamma_i \overline{W}_i Y_i}{D_i^k}}{\sum\limits_{i=1}^{m} \frac{\gamma_i \overline{W}_i}{D_i^k}}$$

where

$$D_i^k = [(X_i - X^k)^2 + (Y_i - Y^k)^2]^{1/2}$$

$$\overline{W}_i = \sum\limits_{j=1}^{n_i} W_{ij}$$

and the initial values X^0 and Y^0 are chosen from

$$X^0 = \frac{\sum\limits_{i=1}^{m} \gamma_i \overline{W}_i X_i}{\sum\limits_{i=1}^{m} \gamma_i \overline{W}_i}$$

$$Y^0 = \frac{\sum\limits_{i=1}^{m} \gamma_i \overline{W}_i Y_i}{\sum\limits_{i=1}^{m} \gamma_i \overline{W}_i}$$

The algorithm stops when for a given number $\epsilon > 0$

$$|X^{k+1} - X^k| < \epsilon$$

and

$$|Y^{k+1} - Y^k| < \epsilon.$$

The convergence of this algorithm has been proven;[12] however, its convergence is very sensitive to the starting values X^0, Y^0 (X_i^0, Y_i^0, for all i in I).

EXAMPLE

Table 1 utilizes hypothetical planning data to locate facilities that will provide five different health services. Service 2, for example, might be pediatrics. Here the institutional policy makers have decided that the population should have a 95 percent chance of being served all of the time. The quantity 1.645 refers to the abscissa associated with the left tail of the standard distribution for the 0.95 probability level. In this instance the population to be served consists of five people located in coordinates (1,1), (1,10), (2,2), (3,3) and (9,3). The cost per mile per service varies from 0 to $4.50 and the expected number of units of service per unit time regardless of whether the time frame is per month or year varies from zero to six visits with a standard deviation of 0 to 0.9.

Table 2 displays the results of the location problem for the five services. In this instance for the five services, we see three unique locations, resulting from the similarity in coordinate points and the pattern of cost per mile of services. If these points and costs were less similar, a pattern of five separate locations would have emerged. The column labeled total services refers to the total services required to fulfill the policy mandate about serving a given population with a given probability. Column 2 (ϵ_i) refers to the accuracy of the location, in this instance we are accurate to two decimal places. The number of iterations is a technical consideration that refers to the efficiency of the computer program.

Table 1 Hypothetical Planning Data

Medical Service i	Probability of Always Being Served α_{ij}	From Normal Tables $G_{\alpha_{ij}}$	Patients' Location X_{ij}	Y_{ij}	Cost per Mile per Service β_{ij}	Expected Number of Units of Service $\mu_{r_{ij}}$	Standard Deviation of Number of Units of Service $\sigma_{r_{ij}}$
1	0.9	1.28	1	1	$8	7	0.3
			1	10	2	3	0.1
			2	2	4.20	4	0.01
			3	3	0	0	0
			9	3	1.20	4	0.2
2	0.95	1.645	1	1	4.50	1	0.9
			1	10	2	2	0.1
			2	2	3.20	6	0.02
			3	3	0	0	0
			9	3	1.30	4	0.3
3	0.9	1.28	1	1	3.30	12	0.01
			1	10	3.00	1	0.1
			2	2	0.50	11	0.03
			3	3	0	0	0
			9	3	4.20	4	0.2
4	0.9	1.28	1	1	0	0	0.54
			1	10	1.40	2	0.1
			2	2	0.75	1	0.04
			3	3	0.20	3	0.02
			9	3	2.40	4	0.3
5	0.95	1.645	1	1	1.52	4	0.3
			1	10	1.20	3	0.1
			2	2	5.00	3	0.05
			3	3	0.30	2	0.01
			9	3	5.10	4	0.2

Table 2 Results of Location Problem for Five Services

Medical Service i	ϵ_i	Location X_i	Location Y_i	Total Service $\overline{W}_i = \sum_{j=1}^{n_i} W_{ij}$	Number of Iterations
1	0.001	1.001	1.001	18.7808	11
2	0.001	2	2	15.17140	6
3	0.001	1.001	1.001	28.43520	17
4	0.001	1.001	1.001	11.28000	3
5	0.001	3.091	2.256	17.08570	63

Table 3 contains the output of Table 2 (location and total amount of service), the average costs per mile per service based on the costs figures in Table 1 and the final result of utilizing the algorithm to solve for a unique location.

DISCUSSION AND FURTHER EXTENSIONS

The necessary conditions for an optimum to (2) subject to (6) provide some insight into the problem.

The Lagrangian expression for the problem given in (2) subject to (6) and (1) is

$$L_i(X_i, Y_i, W_{ij}, \lambda_j) = \sum_{j=1}^{n_i} \beta_{ij} W_{ij} D_{ij} - \sum_{j=1}^{n_i} \lambda_j (W_{ij} - G_{r_{ij}} \sigma_{r_{ij}} + \mu_{r_{ij}}) \quad (14)$$

Table 3 Final Result of Search for Unique Location

Service i	Location X_i	Location Y_i	Cost per Mile per Service γ_i	Total Amount of Services Delivered $\overline{W}_i$
1	1.001	1.001	$3.08	18.7808
2	2	2	$2.20	15.17140
3	1.001	1.001	$2.20	28.43520
4	1.001	1.001	$0.95	11.28000
5	3.091	2.256	$2.62	17.08570

Unique Location	Iterations	ϵ
$X = 1.001$, $Y = 1.000$	3	0.001

The necessary conditions for a minimum are given by

$$\frac{\partial L_i}{\partial X_i} = \sum_{j=1}^{n_i} \beta_{ij} W_{ij} (X_i - X_{ij}) D_{ij}^{-1} \geqslant 0 \qquad i = 1, \ldots, m \qquad (15)$$

$$\frac{\partial L_i}{\partial Y_i} = \sum_{j=1}^{n_i} \beta_{ij} W_{ij} (Y_i - Y_{ij}) D_{ij}^{-1} \geqslant 0 \qquad i = 1, \ldots, m \qquad (16)$$

$$\begin{bmatrix} \dfrac{\partial L_i}{\partial W_{i1}} \\ \vdots \\ \dfrac{\partial L}{\partial W_{in_i}} \end{bmatrix} = \begin{bmatrix} \beta_{i1} D_{i1} - \lambda_1 \\ \vdots \\ \beta_{in_i} D_{in_i} - \lambda_{n_i} \end{bmatrix} \geqslant \begin{bmatrix} 0 \\ \vdots \\ 0 \end{bmatrix} \qquad (17)$$

Inequalities (15) and (16) state that for a given parameter value and a fixed set of W_{ij}, the optimal location for the ith medical service, i in I, has the property that *marginal* changes in either of the coordinate directions yield no change in the objective function.

If λ_j, j in $J(i)$ is interpreted as the imputed value of a delivered service (ith medical service), measured in dollars per service i demanded by the jth patient, then (17) indicates that, at an optimum, the cost of delivering one unit of the medical service to patient j, j in $J(i)$ from the ith medical facility, $\beta_{ij} D_{ij}$ must be greater than or equal to the imputed value of a delivered unit, λ_j, for $j = 1, \ldots, n_i$.

The λ_j do not represent the change in the minimum attainable cost resulting from a "small" change in the associate service demanded r_{ij}, which is the usual origin of the imputed value for a delivered service. Rather, λ_j represents the change in the minimum attainable cost associated with a reduction of one unit in the quantity $[G_{\alpha_{ij}} \sigma_{r_{ij}} + \mu_{r_{ij}}]$. Now it is clear that this quantity can be altered by selecting a different value for α_{ij} and hence $G_{\alpha_{ij}}$, or by altering the estimates of the parameters $\sigma_{r_{ij}}$ and $\mu_{r_{ij}}$ of the probability distribution.

For the moment suppose the administrator of the ith medical service is unconcerned about the variance in r_{ij} and estimates his jth patient's service quality requirement to be satisfied if his actual requirements are met 50 percent of the time. In this instance $\alpha_{ij} = 0.5$ and $G_{\alpha_{ij}} = 0$ and thus $W_{ij} = \mu_{r_{ij}}$. In short, the administration of the ith medical service is only concerned with the first moment of the requirement distribution. In this case, λ_j, measures the change in the minimum attainable cost associated with a small change in $\mu_{r_{ij}}$.

If the administration of the ith medical service feels that the jth patient's demand seeking its services must be met more than 50 percent of the time, then α_{ij} must be set higher than 0.5 which in turn increases $G_{\alpha_{ij}}$ above zero. Then the more undesirable it becomes to fail to meet one of the patient's requirements, the higher α_{ij} and hence $G_{\alpha_{ij}}$ will be set.

For given values of $\mu_{r_{ij}}$ and $\sigma_{r_{ij}}$, the "effective" requirement for patient j seeking service i is $G_{\alpha_{ij}}\sigma_{r_{ij}} + \mu_{r_{ij}}$. The quantity $G_{\alpha_{ij}}T_{r_{ij}}$ can be thought as additional quantity that must be given to patient j, to ensure meeting his requirements with probability of at least α_{ij} over that delivered if only the expected requirement is considered (i.e., when $\alpha_{ij} = 0.5$). A decrease in α_{ij} can be determined so that the value of $G_{\alpha_{ij}}T_{r_{ij}}$ is reduced by one unit. The effect of such a change in α_{ij} on the minimum attainable cost is measured by λ_j. Thus the minimum attainable cost is reduced by λ_j.

NOTES

1. A. Charnes and W. W. Cooper, "Chance-Constrained Programming," *Management Science* 6 (1959): 73.

2. J. Prawda and Arthur P. Hurther, Jr., "A Warehouse Location Problem with Probabilistic Demand," Working Paper Series No. 42, Graduate School of Business Administration, Tulane University, New Orleans, LA 70118.

3. D. J. Bowersox, E. D. Smykar, and F. H. Mossman, *Physical Distribution Management* (New York: Macmillan, 1961), p. 176.

4. J. F. Magee, *Industrial Logistics: Analysis and Management of Physical Supply and Distribution Systems* (New York: McGraw-Hill, 1967).

5. K. B. Haley, "The Siting of Depots," *International Journal of Production Research* 2 (1963).

6. R. C. Vergin and J. D. Rogers, "An Algorithm and Computational Procedure for Locating Economic Facilities," *Management Science* 13 (1967): B-240.

7. T. L. Saaty, *Mathematical Methods of Operations Research* (New York: McGraw-Hill, 1959), pp. 101–103, 106.

8. G. E. P. Box and K. B. Wilson, "On the Experimental Attainment of Optimum Conditions," *Journal of the Royal Statistical Society*, Series B, 13 (1951): 1.

9. A. S. Manne, "Plant Location Under Economics-of-Scale-Decentralization and Computation," *Management Science* 11 (1964): 213.

10. S. H. Brooks, "A Discussion of Random Methods for Seeking Maxima," *Operations Research* 6 (1958): 244.

11. L. Cooper, "Heuristic Methods for Location-Allocation Problems," *SIAM Review* 11 (1964): 37.

12. L. Cooper, "Solutions of Generalized Locational Equilibrium Models," *Journal of Regional Science* 7 (1967): 1.

13. M. A. Efroymson and T. L. Ray, "A Branch-Bound Algorithm for Plant Location," *Operations Research* 14 (1966): 361.

14. J. W. Gavett and N. V. Plyter, "The Optimal Assignment of Facilities to Locations by Branch and Bound," *Operations Research* 14 (1966): 210.

15. R. L. Lawler and D. E. Wood, "Branch-and-Bound Methods: A Survey," *Operations Research* 14 (1966): 21.

16. L. Cooper, "Location-Allocation Problems," *Operations Research* 11 (1963): 331.

17. H. W. Kuhn, "Locational Problems and Mathematical Programming," Colloquium on the Application of Mathematics to Economics. Budapest, 1963. Publishing House of the Hungarian Academy of Sciences, Budapest, 1965.

18. H. W. Kuhn and R. E. Kuenne, "An Efficient Algorithm for the Numerical Solution of the Generalized Weber Problem in Spatial Economics," *Journal of Regional Science* 4 (1962): 21.

19. W. Miehle, "Link-Length Minimization in Networks," *Operations Research* 6 (1958): 232.

20. F. P. Palermo, "A Network Minimization Problem," *IBM Journal of Research and Development* 5 (1961): 335.

21. J. Surkis, "Optimal Warehouse Location." Paper presented to the XIVth International Conference, The Institute of Management Science, Mexico City, Mexico, August 22–26, 1967.

Index